EAT FAT,
BE HEALTHY

*Understanding the HeartStopper Gene
and When a Low-Fat Diet Can Kill You*

Matthew J. Bayan

SCRIBNER

SCRIBNER
1230 Avenue of the Americas
New York, NY 10020
Copyright © 2000 by Matthew J. Bayan

SCRIBNER and design are trademarks of Macmillan Library Reference USA, Inc.,
used under license by Simon & Schuster, the publisher of this work.

DESIGNED BY ERICH HOBBING

Set in Bembo

Manufactured in the United States of America

1   3   5   7   9   10   8   6   4   2

Library of Congress Cataloging-in-Publication Data

Bayan, Matthew J.
Eat fat, be healthy : understanding the heartstopper gene
and when a low-fat diet can kill you / Matthew J. Bayan.
p. cm.
Includes bibliographical references.
1. Coronary heart disease—Genetic aspects.
2. Apolipoproteins—Pathophysiology.
I. Title.
RC685.C6B34 2000
616.1'23042—dc21   99-045721
ISBN 0-684-86527-0

NOTE TO READERS

This book contains the opinions and ideas of its author. It is intended to provide helpful and informative material on the subjects addressed in the book. It is sold with the understanding that the author and publisher are not engaged in rendering medical, health, or any other kind of personal professional services in the book. The reader should consult his or her medical, health, or other competent professional before adopting any of the suggestions in this book or drawing inferences from it.

The author and publisher disclaim all responsibility for any liability, loss, or risk, personal or otherwise, which is incurred as a consequence, directly or indirectly, of the use and application of any of the contents of this book.

This book is dedicated to Dr. Randy Rough, the cardiologist on call at Mercy Hospital in Des Moines the night my heart stopped, May 9, 1996. Over several hours, he pulled me back from death dozens of times. His persistence took me beyond the usual lifesaving measures to a place where the spirit counts for more than the body. I will forever be in his debt.

I am grateful to Dr. Frank Carrea of Reno Heart Physicians and his intrepid lipid nurse, Katie Locke, who together unlocked the real cause of my cardiac problems and set me on the path of fighting the effects of the heart-killer gene. Thanks to Fred and Terry Hinners for referring me to Dr. Carrea.

I can never thank my family enough for the long vigils at my bedside. Beverly, Nicole, and Greg pulled me through as much as any medical procedure. And thanks to Michon, Sam, and Casey for their sacrifices.

Thanks are not enough for my wife, Beverly, for suggesting that I write this book. A year after my heart attack she presented me with the notes she had taken during my hospitalization; these sparked my memory and got me writing.

My appreciation goes to Donna DeGutis for pulling my manuscript out of the slush pile, and to Margret McBride for taking a risk on a first book; to Jake Morrissey for great editing and to Susan Moldow for believing in this project.

This book is also dedicated to those of you who have had a heart attack and to those of you who are trying to avoid one. For anyone interested in improving cardiac health, this book offers suggestions and information I hope will be helpful. And for those of you who carry the killer gene and don't know it, I hope you learn enough to dodge the bullet that's out there waiting for you. I don't want you to have my experience.

Contents

Contents

Foreword

by cardiologist FRANK CARREA, M.D.

A recent article in a national magazine yielded dozens of phone calls from patients. The article talked about how a low-fat diet is not the proper treatment for some heart patients. The article quoted several cardiac researchers and opened the door on the issue of the killer genes discussed in this book. The problem I see is that the article focused so much on how a low-fat diet can be harmful to some heart patients, it created an inadvertent backlash. Many patients don't want to change their diets. They blanch when I tell them they need to cut down on fats and sweets. These resistive patients clutch at any straw to justify their bad eating habits. Consequently, articles that show the dangers of low-fat diets for *some* patients can easily be misinterpreted by the majority of patients, for whom a low-fat diet is essential.

One of my concerns when my heart patient Matthew Bayan told me about *Eat Fat, Be Healthy: Understanding the HeartStopper Gene and When a Low-Fat Diet Can Kill You* was that in showing how a low-fat diet is dangerous for a minority of heart patients, he would be misinterpreted. I feared that heart patients might justify going against the advice of their doctors and face serious health consequences. However, after reading this book, I think *Eat Fat, Be Healthy* does an admirable job of illuminating the differences between these two groups. In simple explanations, Matt walks the reader through the basics of blood chemistry and how the body handles fat. From this he then shows how for most patients the decades-old regimens of exercise, a low-fat diet, and drug therapy have been effective; he then points out the distinctly different therapies needed for carriers of the killer genes he has named HeartStoppers.

When Matt asked me to review and edit *Eat Fat, Be Healthy,* I initially saw my job as checking his science. For the record, I think he effectively describes the disease that caused his heart attack, shows how to detect this disease, and offers treatment solutions. Because the cause of his heart attack only recently became the focus of research, there is much we don't know about the subtle workings of the killer gene. Only a minority of cardiologists have, so far, focused on how to treat patients who carry this genetic disorder. *Eat Fat, Be Healthy* thoroughly examines treatment issues. Though he is not a doctor, Matt has become very knowledgeable about HeartStopper genes because, as he puts it, "My life depends on it."

His case offers hope to others that this disease can be managed effectively. Matt has been my patient for over two years now. When he first visited my office, the composition of his blood cholesterol was not good; he had an abundance of a dangerous form of LDL (bad) cholesterol that put him at risk of another heart attack. Over the past two years we have been able to develop a diet and medication regimen that has reversed his condition. From the standpoint of prevention, I could not ask for better results.

In recent years, science has found that several genes cause heart disease. One popular belief is that if people are overweight and have heart attacks, it's because they didn't take care of themselves; they "cheated" on their diets; they were bad. As we learn more about the genetic causes of heart disease, we understand that this just isn't so. Many people who exercise and eat low-fat diets have heart attacks without warning. More and more we see genetic triggers for these tragedies.

For example, one HeartStopper gene Matt discusses is actually a gene designated as the ApoB gene. This abbreviation stands for apolipoprotein B. It is one of several different genes that cause an abundance of the dangerous form of LDL (bad) cholesterol that caused Matt's heart attack. Another gene, called the ApoE4 gene, also causes production of the same dangerous LDL (known as small-particle LDL). The ApoE4 gene is more obvious than the ApoB gene in its effects; it causes dangerously high cholesterol and triglyceride levels along with obesity. But, as scientists discovered its direct link to heart disease, they also discovered that the ApoE4 gene was a genetic trigger for Alzheimer's disease. Many cardiologists stopped performing the blood test for the ApoE4 gene because of an ethical problem: If they found the ApoE4 gene and confirmed the cause of a patient's heart disease, should they also tell the patient he would develop Alzheimer's? Many patients didn't want to know.

Right now, we know about several genes that cause dangerous levels of small-particle LDL. As research on heart disease continues, I suspect others will be found.

So much for the science. Evaluating it was my original role. However, along the way, I discovered an interesting story in how Matt survived a massive heart attack and how he went from being totally ignorant about heart disease to being quite knowledgeable about what he considers the HeartStopper Effect. He compellingly weaves his personal story into the discussions of the scientific and medical information that in so many books can put the reader to sleep. In one of the oldest tricks in medicine, Matt sugarcoats the pill to make it easier to take. *Eat Fat, Be Healthy* becomes not only an effective self-help book, but also a rather dramatic narrative.

Eat Fat, Be Healthy is entertaining, informative, and on target. I hope you find it as readable and as useful as I did.

Prologue

Have you survived America's greatest killer? Or do you fear you'll someday meet this grim reaper?

Each year, 1.5 million Americans have heart attacks. One-third of them die. Ninety percent of those whose hearts stop before they get to a hospital don't survive. And here's a scarier statistic: roughly half of all heart attack victims have no symptoms to warn them that they have heart disease.

I barely made it to the other side. After hearing my story, a doctor at the American Heart Association said, "You are a very lucky man." I figure that if I could survive an impossible situation on the outer fringe of statistical probabilities, then, forewarned, you can do even better.

Welcome to the other side of death.

We're all on borrowed time. We need to use it well. I hope by chronicling my personal odyssey I can help others avoid the dangers that lurk out there and maybe extend their lives.

For those who have not yet had a heart attack and who have heart disease or high blood pressure or a lousy diet or who smoke, I hope you read closely. *You do not want to experience a heart attack!* It is a horror you must avoid at all costs. Apart from the heart attack's excruciating physical torture that seems as if it will never end, consider that if you survive, your heart will be damaged, your life span shortened, and you won't be able to do many of the things you now take for granted.

Oh, yes. There's another big drawback. The fear that it will happen again. You'll live with it for the rest of your life.

My purpose in this book is to shed light on a little-known, but deadly, genetic condition that strikes down seemingly healthy people. It is a stealthy killer with one purpose: to destroy your heart. Current health screenings frequently overlook the effects of this disease, mistaking it for the more straightforward coronary problems found in the majority of heart disease patients. The traditional treatments for this majority *actually put carriers of HeartStopper genes at greater risk of death* while lulling them into a false sense that they're effectively treating their heart disease.

With the license of a writer and to make this book easier to read, I have named the condition that caused my heart attack the HeartStopper Effect. Several different gene mutations can cause the HeartStopper Effect. The gene that almost did me in is called the ApoB gene, an abbreviation for apolipoprotein B. (Apolipoproteins are a combination of fat and protein the body constructs to move fat through the bloodstream to cells throughout the body.)

The HeartStopper Effect causes two serious problems: *hyperlipidemia,* an abundance of fat compounds such as triglycerides and cholesterol in the blood; and *small-particle LDL syndrome,* which is a proliferation of a particularly sticky type of bad cholesterol that attaches to coronary arteries and builds up quickly.

These problems were actually reported by the American Heart Association in 1965, but only in the past few years have doctors had access to commercial laboratory facilities that could perform the blood tests necessary to screen for its existence.

You may recently have read about Syndrome X, which, among other symptoms, causes hyperlipidemia. Though there are similarities, the HeartStopper Effect is *not* Syndrome X. Syndrome X results from a diabetes-like condition called *insulin resistance* in which body cells don't allow glucose to enter through cell membranes. This results in high blood sugar levels that cause weight gain, high blood pressure, and buildup of arterial plaque. Syndrome X is largely reversible with exercise and diet. Though exercise and diet are important components in treating the HeartStopper Effect, they must be accompanied by drug therapy.

Throughout this book I use my own case history to illustrate the warning signs, diagnosis, and treatment for these deadly genes.

Who can benefit from this book? People who already have heart problems will find out how to determine if they have the

HeartStopper Effect. This is crucial because *the HeartStopper Effect requires different treatment* from most other causes of heart disease. Though I focus on killer genes, heart patients who do not have them can benefit from my discussions of nutrition, drug therapy, exercise, and mental attitude.

Why am I qualified to present this story? Because the Heart-Stopper Effect is such a new challenge, most doctors don't know it exists and they don't know how to treat it. Over the past two years, my cardiologist and I have experimented with various therapies, some fruitful, some damaging. I have been an active participant in the development of my particular treatment, occasionally disagreeing with my cardiologist and suggesting new strategies.

Researchers have found several therapies that counter the HeartStopper Effect, but these treatments must be tailored to the individual needs of each patient. A cookie-cutter approach won't work. Because there is a degree of trial and error in these treatments, I've had to become heavily involved in assessing success or failure and in weighing the risks of each therapy option. In other words, I've had to become an expert; my life is on the line. Only I am in the position to choose what risks I will accept in trying to stay alive.

I've selected topics that show how to integrate what I've learned into a normal routine. I use real situations to illustrate my thinking. I hope you find the stories informative; they're all true.

Eat Fat,
Be Healthy

CHAPTER 1

Borrowed Time

Swimming up through the depths of sleep, I am weighed down by dream and nightmare images. I know something is wrong. The images are not just phantoms of a tired brain, but real demons. They try to suck me back down into a cold, roiling darkness. Some instinct tells me I must fight to the surface of consciousness or die.

I emerge. I know I'm awake, but it still feels like the nightmare. My chest feels crushed by a truck while at the same time it seems to be exploding outward. I'm bathed in sweat and cannot breathe. Only a faint illumination from a streetlamp fights through the blinds of my bedroom. Disoriented and afraid, I turn to see the greenish glow of the bedside clock: 4:00 A.M.

What is happening?

At first I try to calm myself with the thought that I have indigestion. The spicy marinara sauce from dinner had a lot of garlic in it. Could it have affected my stomach? Or do I have food poisoning? No, this is nothing like food poisoning. My stomach does not feel sick. The pain is higher. Heartburn?

No. It is not possible that food could do this. Heartburn. Heart . . .

Oh, my God. Is this a heart attack?

It doesn't seem likely. I've recently had a checkup. And a cardiac stress test. I'm in good physical shape, I exercise every day, I don't eat meat or fatty foods.

It gets worse and now fear sits on my chest as heavily as the pain. I lie still for long minutes, but the crushing pain does not abate. Now I begin to hear and feel my heartbeats. Each one is like a hammer blow to the anvil that is my chest; each one sends the pain ringing through me more and more stridently.

Something I'd read pops into my mind. If it *is* a heart attack, I have to take aspirin. I try to stand, but a white-hot dagger cuts through my body and I land on the bedroom floor on my knees. On all fours I crawl across the carpet and down the hall. Faced with the stairs, I stop. I can't walk down the stairs because I can't stand up. If I try to scuttle down the stairs headfirst, I fear I'll slip and break my neck. I turn around and lower myself a stair at a time, like going down a ladder. My mind is screaming to move faster, but my body can't do any better.

Like a hunchback I scramble into the kitchen and struggle to pull a bottle of aspirin out of a cupboard. Spilling pills all over the counter, I push two tablets into my mouth and then partially fill a glass with water. I wash down the aspirins and fall to the floor, exhausted by the effort.

Emily, my huge Black Labrador–Akita, is whining. She licks at my face, trying vainly to help. She knows something is wrong.

Now I also know something is wrong. Terribly wrong. And I know I have to get out, get to a hospital fast. I am alone. If I pass out, nobody will find me for days. I *must* get out while I still can. Thoughts of indigestion evaporate. I know I am fighting for my life.

Even in my extremity, I think of the dog. I have to put her out so she will not be trapped in the house if I collapse. Crawling now, I make it to the sliding glass door off the dining area, haul it open, and send the bewildered dog into the night. Then I drag myself to the kitchen wall phone and dial 911.

My breath is ragged. It hurts to breathe. Only shallow breaths work. Deeper breaths cause my insides to shatter.

"Hello. This is the 911 operator. How may I help you?"

The voice that scratches from my throat comes as a surprise. I barely recognize it as I quickly spit out my name and address so they will know, just in case. In case I can't go on. I am now struggling for each second of consciousness.

"What do you need?" The voice stays calm, but a little louder. She knows something is bad.

"My chest. Oh, God." A wave of agony smashes through me. I had thought I was in excruciating pain before, but what I had felt so far was as nothing compared to the molten horror that now erupts in my chest. I pray that the old pain will come back. The new pain is beyond belief. I scream as I collapse from my knees to the floor.

"What is it? Sir, what is it? Do you have chest pain?" The operator's voice jumps up the scale and she is now worried. Her professional demeanor slips for a second.

"Help me. Help me." I scream it. I whisper it. It becomes my personal mantra and all I can think of as the seconds crawl by. I am trapped in amber. I know the ambulance will never get to me. I say it over and over again as I writhe on my back. "Help me. Please, help me."

"Sir, try to take steady breaths. Try to stay calm. It will help."

There is no way to stay calm. A freight train is roaring through my chest. And breathing is now a form of torture. I know I have to breathe, but I don't want to.

The smartest thing the operator does comes next. She gives me a goal. "Sir, the ambulance just checked in. They're not far from you now. Just a couple minutes at most. Is your front door locked?"

Knowing the ambulance is near helps me to hang on. There is comfort in knowing I won't be alone in the middle of the night. I can make it a few more minutes. Hell, I could do anything for three minutes.

"I'm opening the door. Be back in a minute."

Now I can barely crawl. Though I've been on my back on the floor for only a few minutes, it feels as if I have gained a hundred pounds. I drag myself across the living room, down the small stairway, across the landing. I think of only one simple task at a time, trying to get each one right, trying not to make a mistake. I flip off the dead bolt and pull the door open, the effort setting off howling agonies in new places in my body. I switch on the front spotlights. One task at a time.

Oh, why didn't I let those people who came door-to-door paint my house numbers on the curb in front of the house? With all the trees and shrubs, what if the ambulance driver doesn't see my house number? What if he drives right by?

I retrace my route and get to the phone, my lifeline. "I'm back." I can't believe the trek I just made.

"How're you doin'?"

"Still here," I gasp.

"Are you lying down?"

"Yes. I'm on the floor," I get out between gritted teeth. Breathing is painful, talking worse.

"The ambulance just turned onto your street. Hang on."

I clutch at the hope that in a few moments, there will be people who can help me. Through the pall of pain, I notice my legs are moving. It is like I'm pumping on a bicycle. I try to stop them, to stay as still as possible, but they have a life of their own. For a few moments I am weirdly fascinated at this disconnection from my legs as I watch them pumping away.

I hear the doorbell and then the storm door opening. "Hello. Where are you?" a voice says.

In a minute, I am surrounded by three West Des Moines EMTs. They get a blood pressure cuff on me. One starts an IV. Questions, voices. I settle into a quiet place in my head, and for a while everything is a blur. The pain is there, but my mind is drifting, my consciousness slipping.

I reorient in the ambulance. Someone is asking me to keep my legs still. "I can't stop them. They're walking all by themselves," I say. I do not know that this is my body's way of compensating for my failing heart by pumping blood with the large muscles in my legs. All I know is it feels better to have my legs pumping, so I don't try to stop them.

I hear the whine of the tires and the steady beat of the big engine. The medics shoot something into me. Lidocaine. I don't feel as bad. Absently, I think of the route we are taking. Six miles. Six minutes. I concentrate on holding on. Then the doors fly open and I am rolling through the darkness of the parking lot, then the light of the emergency room. More scurrying, more controlled chaos.

"Shall we cut your sweats off or pull them off?"

At first the question makes no sense. I blink in the bright light. The nurse wielding the scissors seems eager to use them. "Pull them, please." I have visions of needing my sweatpants to go home in the morning. Optimist.

Then everything goes black.

My heart stops.

At home I had lain in bed five minutes. It had taken ten minutes to get an ambulance. It was another fifteen and I was in the emergency room at Mercy Hospital in Des Moines, Iowa. Half an hour. In that time a third of my heart died. Had I waited another five minutes to call 911, I would have arrested in the ambulance and probably died.

But in the emergency room, they are staffed and equipped for this. Seconds are now crucial. The great survival engine that is the ER revs up, and the staff attacks this body that contains a dying heart. I awake for a few seconds, as if being roused from a nap. Annoyed at the intrusion, I can't figure out why a young nurse is straddling me and pressing on my chest. "What are you doing?" I snap. "Get off me." Then I am out again, returned to a slumber that is not a slumber. I am at the edge, drifting back and forth over the shifting boundary between life and death. I am dancing on a tightrope.

I awake again. The pain is still there, but somehow more distant, removed. It's as if my mind is cocooned in a safe place and my body is somewhere else. There is commotion—another heart attack victim is wheeled into the ER—and staff are trying to keep two stricken men alive. In all the excitement, nobody notices I am awake. A male nurse at the foot of my gurney is complaining to someone, "I can't move him alone. He's bagged. I need help. Somebody has to work the Ambu bag." The Ambu bag is a large plastic football attached to a mouthpiece; by squeezing it, they keep me breathing.

I take off the plastic mouthpiece that covers my lower face and in a jolly voice say, "Here, let me do it."

The male nurse's eyes go wide. "I thought you were out."

"I was. But I'm not now. Where are you trying to take me?"

"The Cath Lab. But we're swamped."

"Hand *me* the bag. I'll do it."

The male nurse looks shocked. "No, I can't let you do that."

"Why not? Some union bullshit?" I'm amazingly lucid and in a frivolous mood. I say, "Look, this is an emergency, right?" The nurse nods. "You need help, right?" The nurse nods again. "And I'm in danger, right?" By now the male nurse is laughing. He's never had a half-dead patient grill him before. "Well, give me the friggin' bag and let's get the hell out of this traffic jam."

With a big grin, the male nurse refits the mouthpiece and puts the blue, translucent Ambu bag into my hands. I squeeze and breathe and we roll out of the ER.

As we roll down a hall, a passing nurse with curly brown hair and a uniform that looks as if she'd bought it from Victoria's Secret comments, "Hey, Jimmy, you guys short on staff?" The male nurse laughs.

I spit out the mouthpiece and in a laughing voice say to the nurse, "Ma'am, this is an emergency. Will you please not distract the driver?" Both nurses laugh because they can't believe it. They are inured to the many strange sights they see in the hospital, but this is beyond their experience.

Then all goes black again. The humorous interlude ends. Over the next three hours, my heart will arrest again and again.

Out of nowhere I hear a male voice say in a matter-of-fact way, "He's dead." His tone is final, solemn.

The voice seems close, but nothing is around me. I am calm, removed from the world, moving into some otherwise, but still connected enough to my body to be able to hear. Part of me is amused. Part of me is alarmed at the meaning of the words I have just heard.

My heart has stopped again.

Someone working on me wants to give up.

My body lies there, the subject of scrutiny, of analysis. People I don't know and will never meet again are deciding my fate. Something about the improbable outcome fascinates me. But my mind can't stay focused. I have a thought and then it is snatched away. I keep trying to return to the important decision these strangers are pondering. I am at the border between life and death. I am trying to understand the interplay of forces and events, but the distractions are enormous. Lights are bursting in battlefield brilliance and I hear explosions, deep and resonant. I am strobing in and out of silence and loud madness, a contrast so large I cannot hold a thought. It happens faster and faster and suddenly I am alone.

Each stoppage of my heart is like a tiny pearl of time suspended in space, strung through by the perfect line of the infinite. Like a ripe grape squeezed in a child's eager fingers, I am squirted out of my body along that line, off into the universe. But it doesn't happen just once. It's as if some cosmic jeweler is stringing a necklace of these events, these places where no-time exists. In each of these pearls is encapsulated a physical transition where my body goes from death to life to death. In between, the crash of two incompatible realities assaults me in a wrenching cacophony of light and sound and cold and heat.

In one of the silences, I see my body with all of its organs and cells going about their specific and complex tasks, all dependent for food and oxygen on the flow of blood over and around them. The engine on which all these cells depend suddenly stops pumping. Oxygen is quickly sucked out of hemoglobin in the bloodstream and consumed by the hungry cells wanting to keep on about their business. Carbon dioxide begins to build up in the blood. Cells begin dying.

To save them, my heart must restart and pump against the inertia of all that blood—pounds of it—that is sitting in my veins preparing to congeal. Those first few pumps will be more difficult than any others as each corpuscle must be bumped along its way from a complete stop.

Electricity shocks my heart and it spasms, sending the first shiver of movement through the arteries and veins and capillaries. It is much like watching a long train of boxcars respond to the first tug of the diesel engine. First one car moves, then the next, and next, as the engine overcomes the inertia of each car and takes up the slack between them. The first cars are moving for several minutes before the last car begins to follow.

Blood cells move, plasma flows, and soon the oxygen-starved

cells of my body are functioning again. Millions of macrophages—the body's tiny repair shops—deploy and locate dead and damaged cells, intent on carrying away the litter of death. Oblivious, the system keeps on about its business at the cellular level, unaware that the consciousness that controls them is far away; unaware that other collections of cells are making decisions that will determine their survival and continued existence.

Then, again, the engine quits, and the little boxcars of food and oxygen bump into each other as they slow down, then stop.

No pulse, no breathing, no movement. It has happened again and the only difference between me and a corpse is my temperature. "He's dead." Is the man who speaks up voicing a consensus or merely his opinion?

Regardless, Dr. Rough, the on-call ER cardiologist at Mercy Hospital, continues his work, stringing the next pearl in my existence.

It is a quiet place, not warm, not cold. In fact, it doesn't seem I have a body at all. I am just here. It is milky white, not bright, just a constant glow all around me. I have been here a long time, yet there is no sense of urgency or desire to leave. Time is meaningless. I am just here in an endless now.

My thoughts clarify and I understand that I am not where I have been all my life. This place is clearly an otherwhere. I sense that the space is infinite and that I can stay forever. Part of me has dim memories of the world I have come from. I remember something about a tunnel of light I am supposed to pass through. But there is no tunnel. There are none of the things I had read about people who had come back from death. I am in something totally different.

I am aware that I have gone over. I have no regrets. I have no fear. It doesn't feel like a bad prospect. It is not something over which I have control, so I accept it in a peacefulness that I have never known. Time goes on. Years, days, minutes. I have been here forever; I have never been born. This is where I had come from, been, and would remain.

Far off there is a tug, a ripple. Something has happened in all the unhappening around me. I am suddenly aware that the other place still exists. The place I had been for a while. The physical place. And I know I can make a choice.

If I concentrate my thoughts on that tug, I can become closer to it. I am not moving, per se, but I can make the ripple, the difference, more accessible. I know that to do so will make me closer to that other place. The physical place. I am curious. I think of the ripple and feel its presence again.

I somehow know that if I bring the ripple closer to my consciousness, it will pull me in. I can see the distortion in the space around me. I know if I enter it, I can go back. If I want to. I ponder this choice for infinity.

It is so easy to go back. Though I like it here, I know that later I will have all of eternity to wander the universe. I feel carefree about returning to the physical world. I know I will be back here again when that interlude is over.

I let the ripple, the force, seep more into my mind. I hear a boom, feel a tug. It is the first thing that has actually happened since I have been in this place. Then I hear a voice coming through the ripple in space and I know I must either sever the connection with the ripple or follow through. I think of my fiancée. She is still over there, in the physical place. Though this floating, infinite otherwhere is comfortable, I remember the flesh, the world of touch and light and sound.

I decide to reenter the world of the so-called real. I want to spend more time with my fiancée because I have not felt or sensed any other living consciousness in the otherplace. The afterlife is not what I had always thought. I am certain that when we are both "dead," we will not be together here, so I want to spend whatever time I can with her before returning to this place. I concentrate on the ripple and feel its tug again.

The boom happens again. Stronger this time. I am almost into the ripple. I have one last chance to turn back.

Far off, a universe away, I hear a voice and I understand what it says.

"Three hundred." I know this is a big jolt of electricity and I know it's headed for me.

Why doesn't the voice say, "Clear"? The voice is supposed to say that.

I actually feel rather than sense the last tug. The voice had come in so distinctly, I know something big is about to happen. Part of me doesn't want to feel what I know I will feel. Birth. Oh, God, maybe I should turn back. Maybe this is a mistake. Then I think of the clear blue of my woman's eyes. I want to look into them again. I let the ripple pull me in.

I am trampled by a raging elephant. It slams me, mauls me, and leaves me gasping. I scream in my head and all the pain I have ever felt is concentrated into one searing second. The assault against my new senses is like the rasp of heavy sandpaper across my brain, my eyes, my eardrums. And it gets worse. Up, up, out of the living guts of a star, I writhe. Through cosmic heat and chaos and an unbearable flash of thermonuclear light, I wrench through the ripple. My own personal Big Bang.

Oh, God, why did I want to do this? Idiot!

With three hundred volts of electricity, they defibrillate me and start my heart for the seventy-second time.

In that moment when I flash from the comfort of where I have been to the bright lights and bustling activity of the Catheterization Lab, there is something familiar. The pain all over, the unfocused, stabbing brilliance of the light, somehow I know these sensations. I have felt them before. It is as if my body holds the memory, not my brain. I cannot think it up; only my body in its agony can offer up these connections from the dim reaches of somatic memory. For a fleeting second I reconnect to my infant self, that searing instant when I left the warm comfort of the womb for the cold, dry universe of independent human existence.

I have somehow short-circuited time. It folds in on itself, and two points, my beginning and my almost-end, are now next to each other with only the tiniest gap to cross. The ends of the long string of my life are brought together and I connect to that far-off point, that memory, and for an instant I am in both places at once, my birth and rebirth.

I am suddenly in the new, cooling universe and the pain is gone.

With the eyes of a newborn I gaze out of my forty-five-year old body.

CHAPTER 2

Trapped

First I heard voices. The deep bass of a male giving orders, the soft female responses. Then a rhythmic beeping. The rustle of cloth against cloth.

At the edges of my vision I saw white-clad forms. One reached over me to someplace above and behind my head. I smelled a faint waft of perfume, the sharp bite of alcohol, the faint odor of bleach. The fluorescent light was bright, but no longer painful.

I recognized that I was in a hospital, but I had no idea why. I remembered the pain, but I did not remember the ambulance ride or waking up or anything earlier than a minute ago.

As I became aware of my surroundings, the horror crept in. I had entered some hideous existential nightmare. I could not move. I was paralyzed. I could not speak because a tube was stuck down my throat.

I am not normally claustrophobic. Small rooms don't bother me. The thought of being tied up in a straitjacket might give me pause. However, there is nothing like being trapped inside your own body to scare the wits out of you.

Terror kicked in when I realized I was drowning and I couldn't tell anyone. Though several people were bustling around me, they seemed painfully oblivious of my being about to choke to death. Everyone had a task and studiously pursued it, all the while acting as if I did not exist.

The only thing I could move was my eyes. I blinked furiously, trying to catch someone's attention. No one looked at me. (I did not realize until later that nobody wanted to look at my face. This was because my eyes were swollen red orbs and my face was terribly bruised from seizures. I looked as if I'd gone twelve rounds with Mike Tyson.)

After my initial efforts to get someone's attention, I focused on the most important thing: getting air into my lungs. It felt as if the airway tube was clogged. By breathing slowly, I was able to draw some air down my throat, around the tube, and some through the tube itself. This went on for hours, breathing shallowly in and out, praying I would not lose the airway. Only my being on pure oxygen made it possible for my lungs to survive on the meager air volume they received.

I had to do something. I panicked as I remembered the ambulance ride. What had happened to me? How long had I been unconscious? Did I have a stroke? Was I paralyzed for life? I had no idea why I was in a hospital. And with ignorance comes fear, wave after wave of it, intensified by my not being able to communicate with anyone.

As I struggled to breathe, frightening images flashed into my mind. I thought of Jimmy Stewart in a wheelchair in *Rear Window,* easy prey to the murderous Raymond Burr. I thought of Stephen Hawking, the brilliant crippled physicist, tapping symbols into a computer to speak in that horrible metallic machine voice. Was I to be like them?

Words flashed through my mind as well. Paraplegic: legs gone. Quadriplegic: legs and arms unusable. So, what was I? I couldn't move *anything*. With grim humor my mind offered up a new word. I was a *totalplegic*.

I struggled to catalog my meager abilities. I could move my eyes to the limits of their orbits. I could blink. Yes, and I could hear. There were voices and the sounds of motion: footsteps, the clink of glass and metal. I heard the steady beep of the monitor above me. Each time I breathed there was a clicking whoosh from whatever machine was connected to the tube that went down my throat.

And smell. That most basic and primitive of senses was cataloging my surroundings. Though my breathing was through my mouth, some slight combination of vacuum and pressure was routing molecules through my nose. The odor of alcohol sliced through the air as a nurse sterilized my IV line and injected a needleful of something. Under the alcohol I smelled the whiff of lilacs. It reminded me of my grandmother. Was this an older nurse? I tucked this suspicion away for when she might enter my field of vision.

I blinked my eyes, hoping that small movement might attract her attention. I endured another defeat as her cushioned footsteps retreated.

Phones rang in the hall. I heard the rattle of wheels as God-knew-what carts or gurneys trundled past the door.

So much activity, yet nobody noticed I was awake. I could have been on the moon for all the attention I was getting. Correction: they were attending to my body, but no one seemed interested in what was happening in my mind. I wanted to scream. I even tried, but the tube down my throat rendered me completely mute.

I could feel that damn tube, big as a subway, reaching down, down in a horrible stiff pillar of discomfort inside me. I could feel the pinch of adhesive tape pulling at the skin of my mouth and nose where the tube was anchored. I could feel a dull, unending pain in my left hand where I remembered the paramedic inserting an IV line in the ambulance. An identical pain was now in my right hand.

Then it hit me. *I could feel.* Pain. Temperature. Pressure.

The weight of the blankets was crimping my toes. A dull, achy pain was all around my eyes and face. And in a flash, the piercing discomfort between my legs resolved itself into a specific sensation and I knew a catheter had been inserted in my bladder.

I could feel.

I pushed back the panic, the frenzy of mental activity I had been in. How long had I been like this? I rolled my eyes toward the far wall where I could just make out the clock. I squinted. Was I reading it right? Had I lain here an hour already?

Under me, along my back, along my legs, I felt the sweat that had poured out of me. The sweat of fear.

But now I had something to think about. How could I have feeling in my extremities if I was paralyzed? This made no sense.

I knew that quadriplegics felt nothing below the neck. What weird variant of paralysis was I experiencing? I could feel but not move? Somehow it seemed an even crueler fate than I had originally imagined.

I searched my brain for anything I knew about this. I flashed back to my college biology courses, tried to remember what I had been taught about nerve synapses, neurotransmitters, and human anatomy. I cursed myself for the homework assignments I had skipped, the lab sessions I had blown off on winter mornings when a trek across the campus tundra could not compete with the warm oblivion of my bed.

How could I receive sensory information through my nerves, but have no motor reflexes? The nerves either worked or they didn't. In my hopelessness a glimmer of hope appeared. Perhaps my paralysis was not permanent?

Again I fought with the tube down my throat. My breath was gurgling now. Somewhere down inside this contraption was fluid. I fought my panic and tried to keep my breathing slow and steady. I learned that the trick was to inhale slowly and keep going until I filled my lungs as much as possible. Then the exhale could be fast. Nothing clogged on the exhale. That precious influx of air was what was so difficult.

I kept at it for a while until I knew I would not drown just yet. The little airway alongside the tube provided enough of a supplement to keep me going. But I had to get someone's attention soon. Having survived whatever assault had felled me, I did not want to suffer the tragic irony of suffocating in a hospital, just feet away from help.

Fear was replaced by anger. I had nothing else to do, so I summoned what energy I had to hammer on the walls of this prison until something broke.

I resolved to move something, anything. I focused on my right index finger. If I could get my hand in motion, I reasoned that I could signal for a pencil and tell these people how I was struggling to breathe. I concentrated grimly on the task of moving just the tip of my right index finger. It seemed like an hour before the finger responded. It twitched slightly. No Olympic gold medalists ever cherished their success more than I did my tiny victory. With that small movement I went from the category of vegetable to animal. Heartened, I kept at it for a long time, finally getting some mobility in my index finger. It was even longer still before someone saw the movement.

The young face and brown eyes of a nurse loomed into my field of vision as she peered into my eyes. I did not smell lilacs. This one carried a far more provocative musky scent. She took my hand and squeezed it. I was able to contract my index finger in only faint response, but it was something. I was elated at this simple, limited human contact. After hours of maddening frustration, I had opened a tiny channel of communication.

To someone else she said, "He's awake."

I squeezed once.

"Can you hear me?"

I squeezed again.

"Can you feel my hand?" She squeezed.

I squeezed once in response.

"I think he hears me."

To me now, "Do you hear me?"

With great exaggeration, I blinked my eyes slowly once. I prayed she would understand I was signaling once for yes, twice for no.

"Do you know your name?"

I squeezed her hand once as I blinked my eyes once.

"He seems lucid," she said.

This went on for several questions before the nurse recognized that one squeeze or blink meant yes, two meant no. When she asked me questions that could not be answered by yes or no, it reminded me of being at the dentist's. Why do dentists always ask you a complex question right after they stick their hands in your mouth?

Slowly, but surely, my right hand began to work. At some point I held it in the universal signal for writing: three fingers together and moving my hand in small circles.

"I think he wants to write."

I felt like Lassie when Timmy's mother invariably said, "I think he's trying to tell us something."

They set a writing pad on my stomach and pushed a pencil into my fist. Someone held my arm in place over the paper. I had thought first grade had been bad on that scary day when we left block letters behind and experimented with cursive writing. I remembered how the paper had shrunk to the size of a postage stamp and the pencil had become like a telephone pole in my untutored hand. With that same feeling of overwhelming ineptness, I tried to form letters on a piece of paper I couldn't even see. My first try was illegible. I rested.

Twenty minutes later, with more mobility in my hand, my second try was barely readable. I wrote, "I'm drowning."

The nurse said, "Everybody feels that way."

I wrote, "No, I am really drowning."

She smiled to humor me, but the expression on her face said that she thought I was only a step above an imbecile on the evolutionary ladder. I kept writing and I kept getting ignored. Having escaped the prison of my body, I was now frozen in the virtual incarceration of hospital procedure. After about an hour of my drowning notes, a nurse performed some kind of suctioning procedure on the breathing apparatus and I was able to get more air through the tube. I still felt as if I were drowning, just not as quickly. My notes were no less insistent. Now I wanted them to take the tube out completely. After a dozen notes, the staff ignored me.

Until Beverly arrived. She was like an avenging spirit. She had flown across half the continent from a conference in Boston to find her fiancé tubed and immobile in Mercy Hospital's intensive care unit in Des Moines, Iowa.

Somehow, I knew the moment she arrived. I had my eyes closed, but I felt her palpable force enter the room. Then her soft blue-gray-green eyes filled my vision and her warm lips kissed my cheek. I felt the first moment of peace since I had awakened. Here was the reason I had come back from death. Each time she touched my face, it felt like the hands of an angel. With the respiration tube down my throat, I could not speak; the first notes I wrote to her said how much I loved having her touch my face. She held my right hand and I squeezed. Now I had a champion.

I wrote to Beverly that I was drowning. She had the nurses look me over carefully.

"Everything seems to be okay here," one of them said. "There's some fluid buildup in his tube that is making him think he's drowning. We just have to clear it out every so often."

I wrote, "Get this thing out."

"Sir, it's too early to take out your tube. You might need it again."

"Then you can put it back in. I don't need it now. Take it out. I really am drowning," I wrote.

Much discussion ensued, Beverly becoming more and more insistent. She had not gotten much sleep and was not in the mood for bureaucratic resistance. God bless her, her actions over the next day probably saved my life.

The lead nurse finally said, "Only a doctor can approve taking him off the ventilator."

By now I could move my whole body. I raised my left arm and crooked my finger for the nurse to come near as my right hand printed out in large block letters, "THEN GO GET A DOC-TOR!" I pushed this note toward her.

After an excruciating wait, a doctor arrived. "You want to be extubated?" he said.

I opened my eyes wide and slowly nodded my head.

"We'll see about that." He motioned the nurses and Beverly into the hall, where an extended conversation took place. I would learn that all major decisions were made in the hall. Several times I heard Beverly's voice growl in a register I had never before heard. She was a lioness defending her injured cub. She had taken my messages with her. The only exchange I heard clearly was when she said, "If he says he's drowning, he's drowning. Look at these, Doctor. He's been writing the same message all day. He's struggling to breathe."

"That's because his lungs are full of fluid, not because of the tube. His heart is weak and his lungs are filling with fluid. Believe me, he needs that tube."

As evening came on, we relented in our battle, too exhausted to continue. Finally, near midnight, Beverly curled up on the reclining chair they had wheeled into my room. Within minutes she stopped talking. I could hear the steady rhythm of her breathing and I knew she was asleep. I envied the soft, easy sounds of her respiration.

I suffered through an endless night of struggling for breath. I was afraid to sleep for fear I would choke while I was unconscious. For long stretches, the only sounds that punctuated the late-night silence of the coronary care unit were the whooshing of my ventilator and the beeping of my heart monitor. I tried not to think. I was suffering from claustrophobia in my own body. I had a tube up my nose, a tube down my throat, a tube in my penis, and IV lines stuck into my hands. I felt violated and hopeless and I began to think of that other place I had been in while I was unconscious.

Why was I struggling? Why had I endured the pain of rebirth? That other place had been problem-free. I realized that I had not even begun to explore its dimensions. It was vast, infinite. It was a universe of unknowns to be learned.

And then I realized I could go back. I could feel the thin border between here . . . and there. I saw how I could make the mental steps and cross the line and be free.

Then a part of me deep inside rose to my consciousness and seemed to grab me by the scruff of the neck. *You wanted to come back here. You wanted to feel a body again. Well, you have what you wanted! Stop yer bellyachin'! If you don't like what's happening to you, then do something about it!*

I was chagrined. How many people had been given not only the choice I had had, but also the means to accomplish it? How many people got to come back?

Yes, I was damaged. But I was making progress. I had been paralyzed and now I could move. I had been thought dead and now I was alive. I resolved to fight one small battle at a time and see where it led. I would not worry about the outcome of the war. I would just fight each minute and let the hours take care of themselves.

I endured the boredom until dawn when Mercy Hospital roused from its slumber. Technicians trundled bulky, rumbling, portable X-ray machines in and out of rooms. Cafeteria workers handed out hot breakfasts that should have been cold and cold breakfasts that should have been hot. Everywhere the staff poked and prodded and examined groggy patients who wanted nothing more than to go back to sleep.

I hadn't slept. I hadn't dreamed. Yet I felt more energetic. I had a purpose. One small fight at a time. I chose my battlefield and arrayed my forces.

"How are you doing this morning?" It was a new shift, a new face. She was in her thirties and moved with the efficiency of experience as she checked my heart monitor and my IV lines.

I wrote on my pad. "I'm still drowning."

Her eyebrows arched in concern. She checked my breathing apparatus and cleared it. "Better?"

I wrote, "For now, but it will clog quickly and I'll have trouble breathing again. I want it out."

Beverly woke up then. Small red lines crisscrossed one side of her face where it had been pressed into the pillow. Her dark hair was askew. I had never seen anyone lovelier. She kissed my forehead.

The nurse said, "He says he's having trouble breathing."

Day two and we were back where we had started. Beverly explained my breathing problem and I supplemented with hastily scrawled notes. Soon we were joined by another nurse. The tempo of conversation picked up. We went over the same ground as the day before.

I couldn't stand it anymore. I thrashed around and wrote in big letters on my pad, "THAT'S IT! GET A DOCTOR. NOW!"

When a doctor arrived, my haggard fiancée allowed no resistance. She didn't even wait to hear the oft-repeated explanations. She took the doctor out into the hall and I heard her insistent whisper: "Look, I'm pulling rank. He wants it. I want it. Now do it."

When she came back into the room, she held me and whispered in my ear, "Hang on, honey. They're going to take it out."

We would learn that nothing, absolutely nothing, happens quickly in a hospital unless it's the result of an emergency code. If your heart hasn't arrested, then you have to let the momentum of the great machine build up. Hours went by as I struggled for each breath. So close to the goal, I morbidly feared that I would choke just short of salvation.

As was so often the case, when action finally came, it was frenetic. First, Beverly and I had to sign forms acknowledging that we understood the risks of what we were requesting, since it was against medical advice. The clipboard disappeared and suddenly I was surrounded by three nurses and a doctor. Tape was removed from my face, hoses were untangled. The doctor said, "When I count to three, blow out hard while we pull out the tube."

He counted. I blew. The bloody apparatus was wrenched out of my chest. I gagged and coughed for ten minutes, but I was able to breathe far better than with the tube. I croaked, "That damn thing was killing me."

Again I got the humoring look. I motioned the doctor closer and in a raspy voice said, "Doc, do you know that when I first came to, I was awake for two hours before anyone noticed me? I was paralyzed and couldn't signal with anything but my eyelids. Nobody told me what had happened to me. Do you have any idea how frightening it is not to know what's wrong with you and to be unable to communicate?"

A look of mild shock passed across his face. I said, "Doc, I don't want to tell you how to run your business, but wouldn't it be a good idea for ICU protocols to include looking at a patient's eyes? And maybe telling everybody that the universal code is one blink for yes and two for no?" From the look in his eyes, I got the sense that someone would get reamed when he got the staff out of my earshot.

I asked him why I had been paralyzed and was surprised to find that my body had not done it itself. He said, "When we did the angioplasty, we had to have you perfectly still. You were thrashing around and seizing, so we used a drug to paralyze you. It's standard procedure."

Medicine is a curious mix of the known and the unknown. When a procedure or medication works for one patient, it is tried on others. If it works most of the time, it becomes standard practice. But then, having become common usage, it is seldom questioned.

Was I drowning? The staff thought I was exaggerating because they had tubed thousands of patients to enable them to breathe. Maybe I was overreacting; I had never been paralyzed before, or tubed. This was my first lesson in the uncertainty that can surround disease, in not knowing where fact leaves off and opinion begins.

It would be several weeks before I would understand that no yellow brick road led to the correct answers. For all their skill and training, the doctors had to grope along a foggy path to the truth. They made educated guesses based on what had worked before.

We would learn in my case that what we thought we knew was not as much as what we didn't know.

CHAPTER 3

Medical Miracles

I am forever amazed at the formerly experimental techniques that have become common practice in cardiac medicine. Five or ten years ago, I probably would have died from my heart attack because the remedies for the sudden, massive blood clot I had formed could not be performed as quickly and efficiently as today. Without surgery and all its attendant preparation, Dr. Randy Rough, the cardiologist who treated me in the wee hours of May 9, 1996, was able to use the latest technology to get to the site of the problem in minutes.

He used an angiogram, a radiologic procedure. With the patient unconscious and purposely paralyzed, the doctor makes an incision into the femoral artery where the leg joins the hip. The femoral is a big artery and provides a highway to the heart. A long, flexible catheter is slipped into this artery and pushed up to the heart. Radioactive dye is pumped up through the catheter so that it will enter the heart. Using X rays, the cardiologist watches on a TV screen as the dye progresses through the heart. Plaque or blood clots can be seen as narrowing or blocking coronary arteries. By moving the X-ray transmitter around the patient's body, doctors can examine the coronary arteries from different angles and get a fairly accurate assessment of the degree and type of coronary blockage.

In my case, all of my cardiac arteries were clear, except for one. The left anterior descending artery (LAD) was completely blocked. This artery feeds much of the front, outside wall of the heart. It is one of the most common arteries to develop plaque buildup, especially in an area where the artery makes a sharp turn. This elbow turn is the site of many blockages. Cardiologists are familiar with it and look there early in their examinations. This turn in the LAD is so commonly the cause of massive, fatal heart attacks that cardiologists refer to it as the Widow Maker. It was the site of my problem.

Once they found my clot, they pumped a stream of urokinase, an enzyme, through the catheter to the site of the clot. Urokinase breaks up clots. Pumping this enzyme directly to the problem spot cleared the clot, and blood could again reach the front wall of my heart. However, this area had been blood-starved for at least forty-five minutes. It would never recover. The damage was irreversible.

Next, the cardiologist inserted a different kind of catheter through the incision in my leg, snaked it up into the LAD, and lined it up with the plaque formation. This procedure is known as angioplasty. At the end of the catheter is a balloon that is inflated to push against the interior walls of an artery and to spread out a plaque formation over a larger area. In my case, what had been a 40 percent blockage was smooshed out to a 10 percent blockage, not enough to affect blood flow. This would reduce the likelihood of another clot's forming.

The incredible thing to me is that during this procedure, my heart kept arresting. Each time it stopped, Dr. Rough charged up the paddles of the defibrillator to three hundred joules and zapped me. Each time, I came back. He said I would become conscious and alert, stay that way for a few minutes as he worked on me, and then I would arrest again.

When heart tissue dies, potassium and other minerals are thrown out of the dying cells. This rapid movement of electrolytes through tissue creates strong electric charges that disrupt the electrical signals for the rest of the heart. It's almost as if, for a short period, the heart and the surrounding tissue function like a battery. An area in or around the heart builds up a charge from the electrolytes moving into or away from it. When the electrical imbalance between the charged area and some neighboring region becomes sufficiently strong, a discharge takes place. These sudden electrical shocks create arrhythmias or worse. In my case, these shocks were so severe, I had seizures that caused me to flail around while I was unconscious. My battered face was the result. When the arrhythmias got severe, my heart stopped beating. Then Dr. Rough would apply a jolt from the defibrillator and start my heart up again. Then the process would repeat.

Not until Dr. Rough was able to open the clot blockage in the LAD did the seizures stop. Whatever cells were still alive in the damaged area of my heart then stopped emitting electrolytes, the electrical imbalances stopped, and my heart began beating with a normal, unaltered rhythm. This electrical disruption was largely the reason that I had to be revived so many times.

I do not remember any of this. I am just amazed that in the middle of a delicate procedure where he was trying to look inside my arteries, moving this sensitive instrument around inside me, pouring chemicals through the probe into my heart, all the while watching the cardiac monitors to see how I was doing, the doctor stops and brings me back to life, then resumes the procedure. Because of the frequent work stoppages to revive me, this procedure dragged on for hours. Because I was in such serious shape, Dr. Rough was meticulous in searching through my entire heart area to be sure there was no other blockage.

So, for a couple of hours, he worked on the clot damage and defibrillated me over fifty times. He was so amazed that I kept coming back, he hung in there and didn't let me slip away.

I asked him later at what point they usually stopped, at what point did they give up on a patient? He said, "If you had been old and feeble, I might have quit. But you were too young for this to be happening to you. You looked strong, and each time your heart stopped, I was able to bring you back. And you were so lucid in between, I just couldn't let you go. As long as you kept coming back, I was going to keep working on you."

When I asked him how many times he had brought me back, he said, "Over fifty. I knew you were in record territory. At the time, I wasn't counting, I was so busy. But when I was done with the angioplasty and looked at the Cath Lab defibrillator readout, I couldn't believe the count. After we had you stabilized, I went out and checked the ER crash cart they had used on you before I got there. The ER crew had revived you twenty-two times. That put the total defibrillations at over seventy-two. I've been a cardiologist over twenty years and I've never seen anything like it. Neither has anyone else I've talked to."

If I had been old, they would not have pushed so far. If I had not responded as well, they would have stopped. If I had not had a persistent cardiologist on call that night, I would not be here. When I think of how Dr. Rough was woken out of a sound sleep and jumped into the fray and did the right things to save me, I am amazed at the luck of the draw.

I could have died in my bed, in the ambulance, in the ER, or on the table in the Catheterization Laboratory. In those couple of hours, any number of things could have gone wrong. During my crisis, any one of several people could have chosen to quit. If any link in that thin, precarious chain of decisions had broken, I would not be alive.

Dr. Rough checked on me several times during my hospital stay and I peppered him with questions about what I had named The Night. While in Mercy Hospital, I was also visited by a few of the ER nurses who had worked on me during The Night. They checked on me every day, amazed at my survival. They told me the staff in the ER were calling me the Miracle Man because they couldn't believe I'd made it. I thanked them profusely. But I never had a chance to thank other nurses and attendants, interns, ambulance drivers, and EMTs. They all did their jobs and went home to bed and most of them had no idea who I was or what happened to me. But they saved me. They carried me through the biggest crisis of my life. I hope some of them by accident pick up this book somewhere, in a bookstore, in a library, in the hospital gift shop. I hope they remember May 9, 1996, and the night the Miracle Man passed through their hands. I thank them. Without them, there would have been no miracle.

CHAPTER 4

Surviving
the Heart-Killer Gene

The ICU nurses paraded into my room with a huge cake, but no candles. They sang "Happy Birthday."

"Where are the candles?" I said.

One of the nurses tapped the plastic line that connected my oxygen mask to the nozzle coming out of the wall. "You're on pure oxygen. You want to go up like a Roman candle?"

This was the first surprise birthday party of my life. Here I was six days after my heart attack, celebrating my forty-sixth birthday with an IV in my arm, a noseful of oxygen, and wired like a Christmas tree. It was not the birthday I had envisioned.

The nurses asked me what I would like as a gift. In my best Colombian accent, I said, "De good drugs. Gif me de good drugs." It was something I frequently said to them. They told me I'd get the good drugs later if I was good. We compromised on something I truly did want: a new urinal. The original was getting a bit rank.

With a flourish, one of the nurses brought a new plastic urinal from supplies and used a Magic Marker to print my name and "Happy Birthday" on it.

"Use it! Use it!" they chanted. I almost took them up on it right then, but even I, who was "difficult," had limits.

They cut the cake and everyone started eating. When my piece got to me, I asked, "Is this fat-free?" I had already been indoctrinated by the nutrition staff.

One of the nurses said, "No, this is *real* cake." She was a sweet woman, but she looked as if she had been eating real cake about a decade too long.

"Are you trying to kill me?" I took a mouthful for ceremony, but I was already scared to death of fat and sugar.

Looking back, I realize how many incidents occurred that were wildly contradictory. I was in a top-notch cardiac unit where the dietitians counseled me on the need for a low-fat diet, yet the ICU nurses gave me cake. It was no less crazy than the food menus I filled out each morning. On them were items like Salisbury steak au jus. *Au jus* means, basically, we're talking about hamburger floating in its own grease. And this is on a menu with the heading "Heart Healthy."

I decided to have some fun with the nurses after they left. I used the intercom on my bed to call the nurses' station. "Do you have any more matches out there? I ran out."

"What?" was the strident reply from the charge nurse.

"Matches. You know. My family wanted to actually have some candles on the rest of the cake. It's just not a birthday without blowing out the candles."

"Don't you move!"

In exactly seven seconds, three nurses ran into my room, one carrying a fire extinguisher. They immediately saw that we had no candles burning. The first nurse squinted her eyes. In a mock-threatening voice, she said, "You'll pay for this."

They all laughed and left the room. My mother, who had once worked in a hospital, looked at me gravely and said, "You keep playing with them, they'll get you."

They did. That night, when they brought "de good drugs" to help me sleep, they also gave me a shot of Lasix without telling me. Lasix is a diuretic that begins to squeeze the fluids out of you almost immediately. Within twenty minutes, I urinated a river. And this went on all night. It's a special little revenge nurses have for their "difficult" patients.

It kept me up all night. In the prank wars, I was now seriously behind.

I have survived more than three years. *Survived* feels like the wrong word because my health is in sharp contrast to the weak, fragile creature I was on my forty-sixth birthday. I'm in better physical shape now than I was before my heart attack. But the journey from there to here was made of many small steps.

I look back on that birthday in the hospital as a turning point. It was the moment when I began to look suspiciously at everything I ate. I had over twenty years of experience in the field of nutrition, but eating suddenly became a life-and-death experience, something to analyze as if I were starting from scratch. I was motivated to read medical journals and research papers, to question my cardiologist about topics he had never before had to explain to a patient.

Saying no to a piece of birthday cake set me on a path of discovery through the realms of blood chemistry, genetics, cardiology, and therapeutic nutrition. I had to relearn all I had thought was fact about "good" and "bad" foods. My killer gene had changed the rules.

There is much more detail to explore for those who are interested in the chemical and physiological aspects of this disease, but my purpose here is to explain the basic concept of what the HeartStopper Effect is and how it goes about the insidious task of killing its hosts. I want to help you identify whether you have this disease so you can do something about it before it's too late.

The whole story revolves around fat. The human body ingests fat, manufactures fat, burns and stores fat; it distributes and redistributes fat every day. In normal people, this process follows predictable paths. The normal body is fairly adept at fat management. The genes that cause the HeartStopper Effect disrupt this fat management and distort blood chemistry so that fat is deposited in coronary arteries as cholesterol plaque. This plaque can build up incredibly fast. It can endanger even seemingly healthy adults.

Picture this: male, aged forty-five, six feet two inches, two hundred pounds, exercises every day, never smoked, rarely eats meat, has a low-fat diet, has low job stress. That was me.

Why, then, did I wake up from a sound sleep with a massive heart attack, a myocardial infarction (MI) caused by blockage of one of the arteries that feed the heart? There were clues. My father died of an MI at fifty, my grandfather at fifty-seven. But they both ate high-fat diets and, at least in the case of my father, had high stress right before the MI. In contrast, there seemed no apparent cause for my heart attack.

First, let's look at how cholesterol plaque can cause an MI.

CHOLESTEROL PLAQUE

Cholesterol is a complex lipid or fat compound. Cholesterol does not float through the blood all by itself. To move around in the body, it must be linked to protein, hence the term *lipoprotein*. This package of protein and fat moves through the blood to supply cells with fat. In a normal transaction, a lipoprotein bumps up against a cell's outer membrane and the cell absorbs the fat. However, for someone with the HeartStopper Effect, the lipoprotein we call apolipoprotein B, for instance, does not perform in a normal way. ApoB moves into arterial walls 40 percent faster than other lipoproteins. Once there, it is more likely to create dangerous, unstable plaque.

What is this stuff called plaque? How does it form? Where does it come from?

Visualize a tube narrower than your little finger. Blood passes through that tube called a coronary artery to feed the heart muscle so it can pump blood to the rest of the body as well as itself. Over time, tiny particles of cholesterol in the blood stick to the walls of the artery. These particles build up into what is called cholesterol plaque.

It appears we live almost all of our lives with plaque. Autopsies show that cholesterol plaque is found even in children. For the normal individual, this plaque builds slowly over decades, but never reaches a thickness sufficient to block an artery. For those who develop heart disease, the plaque grows more substantially, but also usually at a steady pace. For those with developing heart disease, this plaque thickens and eventually begins to block the flow of blood through the artery, causing *angina pectoris,* chest pain. Angina usually starts in one's late fifties and is usually brought on by exertion. If insufficient blood flows through one of the arteries to the heart, the part of the heart that is fed by that artery begins to get starved for oxygen. If the afflicted person relaxes and reduces the load on the heart, the pain goes away. For those with chronic angina, a prescription of nitroglycerin is used to provide temporary relief by causing coronary arteries to dilate, allowing more blood to flow. Other symptoms of clogged arteries are shortness of breath and dizziness.

If the plaque blockage of an artery increases to where the artery cannot carry sufficient blood to the heart for a prolonged period, that part of the heart fed by the blocked artery begins to die. This is a heart attack. In normal heart disease cases, angina symptoms usually start slowly and increase over time, giving warnings along the way.

By the time we are adults, almost every person has some arterial plaque. Such blockage is not considered serious until it reaches approximately 70 percent closure of the artery. Prior to that, there is sufficient blood to supply the heart's needs, even during exercise. However, with blockage above 70 percent, the flow of blood is too restricted; the heart muscle becomes oxygen-starved and pain results. Eventually, total blockage can occur.

Depending on which artery or arteries this blockage occurs in, the impact on the heart will vary. Total blockage of some of the minor arteries can cause discomfort or mild heart attacks, but afterward, the patient is able to function fairly normally. In my case, the artery being blocked was a crucial one—the left anterior descending artery (called the LAD), definitely not one you can easily live without. It feeds the front wall of the left ventricle, the part of the heart that gives blood the final big push as it leaves the heart.

Doctors now have options for treating arterial blockage, the most common being angioplasty and, for advanced cases, coronary bypass surgery.

After the angioplasty balloon pushes the cholesterol plaque against the arterial wall, the site of the original blockage may not continue to stay clear. In about a third of angioplasty cases, the artery does not respond well to being stretched outward. It constricts again to its previous shape, usually within a few months. Doctors will then recommend insertion of a *stent* to keep the artery open. A stent is a small stiff tube made of a screenlike material. Its support inside the artery keeps the artery from closing down. It sounds crude, but it works.

With angioplasty and stents, all the surgical work is done inside the body using various tools that are worked into place within coronary arteries through incisions in the femoral arteries in one's legs. Bypass surgery, however, is major surgery. The chest is "cracked" by cutting open the sternum and spreading apart one's ribs. The heart is exposed. Surgeons construct detours around clogged sections of coronary arteries by sewing in segments of veins they have cut from elsewhere (usually the patient's legs). After coronary bypass surgery, it takes months for the patient's wounds to heal and for bones in the chest to knit.

The problem with these approaches is that if the patient does not have a healthy diet and does not change behavior, plaque will continue to grow, and eventually these same sites will clog again, along with new sites. How often do you want your chest cracked? How often can you survive major surgery?

For most people, arterial blockage occurs over a long time and never exceeds 70 percent. They go their whole lives without heart problems. Plenty of people on high-fat, high-sugar diets are couch potatoes, smoke, and have high-stress jobs, yet they never get angina and never have a heart attack.

Then there's the group that has the HeartStopper Effect. Recent research shows that roughly 25 to 30 percent of adults carry HeartStopper genes. Genetic mutations that negatively affect blood chemistry are evident in 80 percent of patients with coronary artery disease. For us, there is no long, gradual buildup of plaque into our sixties and seventies. For us, the timetable is accelerated; plaque can build at an alarming rate, regardless of our stress levels, our diets, or our physical conditioning. For us, the tiny particles of cholesterol are abundant and sticky. They cling to arteries in a mad race to destroy us. And for us, there is an added twist. We don't grow the same plaque as everybody else.

STABLE AND UNSTABLE PLAQUE

In a normal individual, stable plaque builds up slowly and becomes a danger only when it threatens to close down a coronary artery. Unstable plaque, on the other hand, is dangerous no matter how much of it is present because it has the potential to tear and create a sudden blood clot.

These different characteristics of plaque are determined by the amount and type of cholesterol floating in the blood. In simple terms, when blood triglyceride and LDL cholesterol levels are high, plaque is gooey and unstable as it grows. When blood triglyceride and LDL cholesterol levels are low, the plaque becomes tougher, less mobile.

How can we deal with this? If we starve unstable plaque of its building blocks, it shrinks against the artery walls. It tightens up and becomes tougher. It is far less likely to rupture.

So, to treat the effects of the killer genes, it's necessary to deal not only with the existence of plaque, but also its composition.

All plaque is a combination of fats and proteins that create a new interior wall inside an artery. A fibrous protein cap grows over the surface of stable plaque and holds it together. Stable plaque is the type of plaque that both normal individuals as well as the majority of heart disease patients grow.

Unstable plaque grows more quickly. The fibrous cap that grows over and protects normal plaque is not fully present in unstable plaque, leaving it open to damage. Think of the difference in consistency between peanut butter and honey. Stable plaque is more like peanut butter; unstable plaque is more like honey. Unstable plaque is more susceptible to movement of the body, to blood pressure changes, and to changes in the volume of blood passing through the artery. Pieces of unstable plaque can break off; it can crack or rip. This is because it is less tough than stable plaque and because the protective protein cap is only partially present or not present at all.

When unstable plaque rips or cracks, the blood senses a break in the blood vessel; it clots at the scene of the wound. However, in this case there is no wound, no breakage in the artery; there is only a breakage in the plaque wall. A small clot usually forms, breaks down, and dissolves without blocking an artery. However, a big tear can cause a big clot and a sudden, totally unexpected heart attack.

And guess what? When unstable plaque is involved, a heart attack can occur long before blockage of a cardiac artery reaches 70 percent, long before there is any warning from chest pain.

How can this happen?

Take my case. Dr. Rough used an angiogram to actually look at my arteries from the outside through the use of real-time X rays. The artery that caused my heart attack was totally blocked. Not by plaque, but by a blood clot. Once he cleared the clot, he saw that the original plaque blockage was only about 40 percent, not enough to cause an MI or the warning of chest pain.

So, what had happened? The consensus in my case is that the unstable plaque coating on the walls of the artery actually ripped as a piece of plaque broke free. Blood platelets passing over the site interpreted this as a break in the wall of the artery and began clotting to repair the breakage. The clotting continued until the artery was totally blocked and the MI resulted.

The good news is that it's possible to manage this deadly plaque. The bad news is that first you have to know you have the problem. Let's look at the basic mechanisms that are manipulated by this disease as it forms unstable plaque.

CHOLESTEROL

Cholesterol is a building-block molecule that the body uses to produce all sorts of other substances such as vitamin D and steroids. We've all heard of steroids in reference to muscle building in athletes. But many more steroids are produced in our bodies, all made from cholesterol. For example, three of the most important human steroids are testosterone, the male sex hormone; progesterone, a female sex hormone; and estrogen, the hormone that regulates a woman's reproductive cycle. Without these three steroids there would be no sex drive, no sex, and no reproduction. The human race would perish if we could truly become cholesterol free. So, the advertising media's campaign to make us think we need to eliminate cholesterol is misinformation.

We're inundated with information about cholesterol all the time. It's become conventional wisdom to limit our intake of cholesterol. Almost every food package now shows the cholesterol content per serving to help us in this task. But what's important about cholesterol is not so much the amounts in the foods we eat as how much of it winds up in our bloodstreams.

Cholesterol is a fat compound that we can ingest or that our bodies can produce. You can starve your body for fat—eat no fat at all—and you will still have cholesterol in your blood. The human body is a complex chemistry set. It will break down carbohydrates and proteins and build cholesterol from the ground up if it has to. We cannot stop this process.

Considering the media bombardment of the past two decades, cholesterol has become equal to kryptonite in our perceptions. We hear terms like "good" cholesterol and "bad" cholesterol as we strive to exclude *all* cholesterol from our diets and our bodies. But cholesterol is not an optional food ingredient. It is an essential component basic to the functioning of the human body.

There are two main types of cholesterol: good and bad. The good cholesterol is called HDL for high density lipoproteins; the bad cholesterol is LDL for low density lipoproteins. (A lipid is a fatty acid; it is the building block of more complex forms of fat. Where you see *lipid,* just think "simple fat." When a lipid is attached to a protein, it is called a lipoprotein.)

HDLs and LDLs engage in a constant tug-of-war within our bodies. The low density lipids are the dangerous ones that attach themselves to the walls of arteries, build up, and choke off the blood flow. This causes chest pain and eventually a heart attack. The high density lipids are the beneficial ones; they actually go out and "grab" LDL particles and carry them away from artery walls and back to the liver for disposal. They are like scrubbers. They keep the arterial system clean. Otherwise, we'd all clog up rather quickly.

For a healthy heart and circulation system, HDLs and LDLs

must be in balance. There must be enough HDLs to keep the LDLs under control. The killing mechanism of the Heart-Stopper Effect is to throw off this balance—to allow the LDLs to overcome the HDLs and to build up unstable plaque in coronary arteries.

How does the gene do this? Another brief chemistry lesson. LDLs come in three forms: large-particle, intermediate-particle, and small-particle. Large LDL particles are easy for the HDLs, the scrubbers, to grab and to move around. It's the small-particle LDLs that are dangerous. HDLs have a tough time grabbing them. (It's like the difference between catching a softball versus a golf ball.) Consequently, the small particles build up in coronary arteries almost unimpeded. The HeartStopper Effect stimulates the body to produce more small-particle LDLs. Then, to be extra lethal, it also suppresses production of HDLs. So, not only does the HeartStopper Effect load up the body with the worst building blocks for unstable plaque, it also reduces the body's ability to move these building blocks away from artery walls. Double whammy.

TRIGLYCERIDES

Triglycerides are simple fatty molecules. They are like building blocks for other, more complex fat compounds such as cholesterol. Unlike cholesterol, which takes weeks and months to increase or decrease in the body, triglycerides increase or decrease in a matter of days. Their existence in the blood is very much influenced by sugar and alcohol consumption.

Triglycerides play the trigger role in crossing over from large-particle LDL production to small-particle production. When triglycerides are abundant in the bloodstream, they provide the building blocks the HeartStopper needs to increase small-particle production. This crossover point appears to be when triglycerides exceed 140 to 160 mg/dL. (All of these measurements are in milligrams per deciliter, so from now on I will drop the mg/dL designation.) If one produces large amounts of small-particle LDL, one is classified *LDL Type B* or *LDL Subpattern B*; if one produces mostly large-particle LDL, one is classified as *Type A* or *Subpattern A* (normal); one who produces both is *Intermediate*. Generally, in normal individuals the production of small-particle LDL is less than 15 percent of total LDL. In carriers of a killer gene, small-particle LDL production can rise to 35 percent, 40 percent, and higher. *Being Type B all by itself constitutes a threefold heart risk.*

Because triglyceride levels can fluctuate rapidly, it does not take much candy and brownies or alcohol or fast-food bingeing to cross over into small-particle production. This crossover can happen in a matter of days.

Triglyceride levels in the blood directly affect the production of LDLs. High triglyceride levels increase production of LDLs, low triglyceride levels decrease production. One can see that managing triglyceride levels not only affects total LDL production, but also is effective in managing the Type A/Type B crossover. Diet and drug therapy can beneficially use this crossover point.

So, theoretically, by starving the body of triglycerides, by staying below the crossover point, we should be able to decrease the building blocks necessary for small-particle LDL production. In normal people this is true. The problem is that for those of us afflicted with the HeartStopper Effect, triglyceride levels tend to stay high, no matter what we eat.

What It Means

So, now we have seen that cholesterol comes in two flavors: HDL and LDL. We've seen that LDL can be small-, medium-, or large-particle. We've seen that plaque can be either stable or unstable. And we've seen that triglycerides are the enablers that affect small-particle LDL production. What do we do with this information?

Unfortunately, we have been conditioned over the past two decades to look at cholesterol simplistically. When we get tested for blood cholesterol levels, we're usually given total cholesterol counts. This is misleading for those with a heart-killer gene.

Total cholesterol measures just that, all the cholesterol in the blood. It does not distinguish between HDL and LDL levels. The American Heart Association and most doctors will counsel that a total cholesterol level under 200 is best. Over 200 is riskier as the level rises. It is generally accepted that as the level approaches 300 or higher, one is in great danger.

However, if we only use total cholesterol as our indicator (as is the case in general health checkups given by general practitioners), we are completely uninformed about the existence of the HeartStopper Effect. For example, someone could have a cholesterol of 200 and be told by his doctor he's in great shape. But he could have a high small-particle LDL count and his body could be building up arterial plaque at a hellacious rate. He leaves the doctor's office feeling confident, and six months later he's dead. This is more likely than you might think; 80 percent of people with coronary artery disease *do not have elevated cholesterol levels.* So, a total cholesterol count is only effective in finding an abnormally high cholesterol level, which requires immediate treatment; it is virtually worthless as a diagnostic for many people with either straightforward heart disease or the HeartStopper Effect. How many people leave their doctor's office certain that they are okay, when in fact they carry the seeds of sudden death in their chests?

The first step to finding out if you have the HeartStopper Effect or any other kind of coronary artery disease is to get what's called a lipid panel. Unfortunately, most doctors usually don't order this test unless one's total cholesterol is already high. This blood test breaks down total cholesterol and shows HDL and LDL levels as well as triglyceride levels. These are essential numbers for *beginning* diagnosis only, because even a lipid panel is not a conclusive indicator for carriers of a HeartStopper gene. Many carriers have lipid panel results that are completely normal, completely misleading about what is going on deeper down in their blood chemistry. But let's use the lipid panel for now because it is cheap, widely available, and is valuable for managing health status in other types of heart disease patients and in the population in general.

Let's use the above example again. A forty-year-old man has a total cholesterol of 200. But his HDL is 30 and his LDL is 170. His triglyceride level is 250. His HDL is too low to stop plaque buildup. The ratio of HDL to total cholesterol is 6.7 (divide total cholesterol by HDL), a time bomb.

But remember, his total cholesterol is 200, within the commonly accepted healthy range. If we relied only on a test of total cholesterol, we would miss the underlying problem completely.

To be clear, for most people concerned about their health, a total cholesterol level under 200 is usually considered healthy. By far, this is the majority. But how do you know if you are part of the "normal" majority or a carrier of a heart-killer gene? If you have the HeartStopper Effect, ignorance can be fatal.

Knowledge of the HeartStopper Effect is actually quite advanced. Viable treatments exist. The problem is that many cardiologists are not primed to look for the special genetic signals. In the great wave of heart patients that washes over doctors every year, it's tough to spot those who have killer genes versus those who have bad blood chemistry because of lousy diets, lack of exercise, and too much alcohol, stress, and smoking.

Those of us who carry these genes get lumped in with the rest. This is dangerous. I'm an example of how this can happen.

Following my heart attack, my doctors highly recommended that I enroll in a course of treatment developed by Dr. Dean Ornish. This treatment plan consists of three elements: radically low-fat diet, stress management and promotion of emotional well-being, and aerobic exercise. In all, it's a well-thought-out plan of treatment. Dr. Ornish has achieved some startling reversals of cardiac artery blockage. He has turned the conventional wisdom about heart disease treatment on its ear.

The most controversial part of what has become known as the Ornish Diet is its nearly no-fat basis. For many patients, this is a difficult bridge to cross, but for those who make it, eating almost no fat becomes a religion. These folks are the Greenpeace of the cardiac community.

I tried the Ornish Diet and I think it has merit for the majority of cardiac patients. The problem was that in my case it could have proven to be dangerous. Killer genes and a no-fat diet don't mix. On the surface, this seems illogical, inconsistent. If fat causes cholesterol and cholesterol builds up as arterial plaque, then cutting off the source of the problem should solve the problem, right? Not so fast.

First of all, the body must have cholesterol to function. The body manufactures cholesterol no matter what we eat. It's the quantity and composition of the cholesterol that are important.

But remember: successful treatment of the HeartStopper Effect rests on the need to keep HDL levels high and to keep the body from creating small-particle LDLs.

For someone with the HeartStopper Effect, cutting out all or almost all fat from the diet causes the body to look for energy elsewhere. After all, the body has only three sources of energy and material: fats, proteins, and carbohydrates. If we take away fats, the body must find fat-building blocks in proteins and carbohydrates. My firsthand experience with this phenomenon came when I restricted my fat intake to less than ten grams per day. An ultra-low-fat diet for me could have been thirty grams of fat, so I was really being extreme. This was soon after my heart attack. My cardiologist at the time did not know I carried a killer gene. He was perplexed that on such a fat-restricted diet, my LDLs and triglycerides were rising. This was a counterintuitive result.

Several months later, after I consulted with a new cardiologist, he and his assistant finally determined that my body's chemistry was doing an end run around my low-fat, low-sugar diet. My body was converting the carbohydrates that were now abundant as fat replacements in my diet—oatmeal, corn, pasta—into sugars. This drove up my triglyceride levels, which allowed the killer gene to manufacture LDLs. By whatever means it took, this enemy gene was determined to clog my arteries and kill me.

Although he felt that the Ornish Diet was good therapy for most cardiac patients, my cardiologist did not feel that Ornish's approach was good for me or for those who have the HeartStopper Effect. Ornish's approach attempts to correct coro-

Receive **2 FREE Gifts**

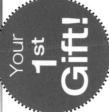

Your
1st
Gift!

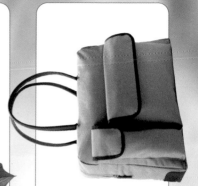

Your
2nd
Gift!

see details inside.

Your FREE
Flower Petal
Umbrella

FREE
when you order

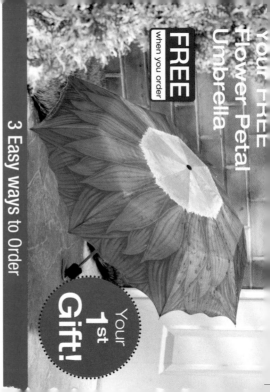

Your
1st
Gift!

3 Easy ways to Order

 BY MAIL:

Yves Rocher Inc.
P.O. Box 1001, STN A
Longueuil, QC J4G 2T4

 BY PHONE:

Order Toll-FREE
1-800-361-2746

 BY WEB:

www.yvesrocher.ca

See all the details on how you can receive your FREE gifts on pages 4-5.

nary artery disease through nutrition and tries to avoid drugs unless absolutely necessary. Though I agreed with the philosophy of the Ornish Diet, I could not follow it. To illustrate, my triglycerides pre-Ornish were around 178—moderately high; after a month on the Ornish Diet, my triglycerides shot up to an extremely high 415! Rather than using the ultra-low-fat approach of Ornish, I needed to augment my dieting efforts with cholesterol-lowering drugs and—pure sacrilege to Ornish—*increased fat intake.* My enemy was just too strong, too wily, too treacherous.

I am not alone in having an unexpected response to a low-fat diet. This seeming anomaly is further illustrated in a 1994 study conducted by the Lawrence Berkeley Laboratory at the University of California. The study was designed to show the effects of a high-fat diet versus a low-fat diet on blood lipid levels. The study focused specifically on how diet affects individuals with normal levels of small LDL particles (Type A) compared to those with high levels of small LDL particles (Type B). Going from a high-fat diet to a low-fat diet lowered total cholesterol, HDL, LDL, and triglycerides for test subjects, but there was one unexpected result: none of the Type B subjects converted to Type A, but in the six-week period of the test, *41 percent of the Type A group converted to Type B when they went on a low-fat diet* (in this case, 24 percent of calories). Also, the drop in protective HDL for this converted group was greater than in the Type A subjects who remained Type A.

These results were on a diet with 24 percent of calories coming from fat. I would call such a diet moderately low-fat. It's when you get down below 10 percent of calories that you have a really low-fat diet. The Ornish Diet recommends fat intake of 10 percent of caloric intake.

If 41 percent of a randomly selected test group developed the dangerous small-particle LDL syndrome by adopting a diet change that definitely was not drastic, how can cardiologists and nutritionists routinely recommend major reductions in fat intake without much more detailed analysis of a patient's condition?

To really nail down this issue, consider this: The same University of California researchers repeated their study and reported findings in 1999. Instead of using a fat intake of 24 percent of calories as in the original study, they reduced fat intake to 10 percent of calories. In this study, *32 percent of the male subjects converted from normal Type A to the dangerous Type B LDL subclass in only ten days.*

So, what if you're not under a doctor's care, are not at particular risk of heart disease, but just want to shed some extra pounds? Assuming your LDL is the normal Type A subclass, your new diet could convert you from normal risk to a triple heart attack risk in from ten days to six weeks. Without the diagnostic information provided by an LDL subclass test, you face huge risks even when you think you're doing something good.

To be clear: If you reduce fat intake, it is unavoidable to increase carbohydrate intake. The type of carbohydrates you eat have a large effect on the amount of triglycerides and small-particle LDL your body will produce. Cake, cookies, candy, and other sugar-rich foods will cause a rapid increase in triglycerides, whereas vegetables, fruits, and grains won't.

Depending on your fat intake, *any* carbohydrate, whether simple or complex, can be converted to triglycerides and then to small-particle LDL. Carriers of a HeartStopper gene can counteract this process (a) by not adopting an ultra-low-fat diet; (b) by starting a doctor-supervised drug regimen; and (c) by keeping consumption of saturated fats as low as possible (and always below 7 percent of total calories).

It is essential for doctors to diagnose and treat each individual *as an individual,* rather than relying on the one-size-fits-all treatment paradigm that has for so long dominated cardiology and nutrition. It also shows that LDL subclass testing is essential for proper diagnosis and treatment of coronary artery disease.

Recent population studies show that 30 to 35 percent of adult males and 17 to 20 percent of adult females have small-particle LDL syndrome. These are numbers that cannot be ignored if proper, ethical care is to be given.

LIPID PANELS

The interactions of total cholesterol, HDL/LDL mix, and trigly-cerides may seem complex. But the whole mix is manageable if one remembers some general rules.

Most doctors would recommend that total cholesterol should be under 200; closer to 150 would be better. Second, HDL should be around 45 or above for males, 55 or above for females; LDLs should be in the low 100s, preferably under 100. Third, triglycerides should be under 140 for most people; for heart patients, under 100.

Can you be above or below these numbers? Yes. These are targets, not absolutes. Probably the single most important number is the HDL level. Below 45 is not good. Above 50 for males and 60 for females seems to have a protective effect far beyond what one would expect. Recent research has shown that people with high HDL levels (70–90 range) can have high cholesterol and yet do not seem to be prone to heart disease and tend to live into their nineties.

People with the HeartStopper Effect will not naturally have high HDL levels. So, if you've recently had your cholesterol checked and you have very high HDLs, chances are that you are not going to have significant plaque buildup. You probably don't have a heart-killer gene.

To give you a reference point, here were my numbers five weeks before the heart attack; five weeks after the heart attack; and almost nine months later. (Note: all readings are in milligrams/deciliter of blood [mg/dL].)

MY BLOOD VALUES 5 WEEKS BEFORE HEART ATTACK (3/31/96)

Total Cholesterol	High Density Lipoproteins (HDL)	Low Density Lipoproteins (LDL)	Triglycerides
258	43	169	172

Cholesterol/HDL ratio = 6:1 (risky)

On the surface, these values don't seem too out of whack. Most labs would consider my LDL and triglycerides within their range for normal patients. The total cholesterol of 258 is considered high, but not dangerously high. Yet in my case, the above values were a formula for disaster. Look at the ratio of total cholesterol to HDL. At 6:1, my risk of heart attack was two to three times normal. My family history of hyperlipidemia quadrupled my risk all by itself. So, just before my heart attack, my likelihood of having a heart attack was increased roughly six times normal from these two factors alone. I would later find that my small-particle LDL production added in another threefold increase in risk. I had *nine times* the normal person's heart attack risk!

MY BLOOD VALUES ON THE ORNISH DIET (6/17/96)

Total Cholesterol	High Density Lipoproteins (HDL)	Low Density Lipoproteins (LDL)	Triglycerides
203	26	94	415

Cholesterol/HDL ratio = 7.8:1 (high risk)

Even though my total cholesterol has dropped 55 points, my protective HDL has also dropped dramatically. My cholesterol/HDL ratio is worse. The doctor who was treating me at the time was pleased with these numbers because my total cholesterol had come down significantly. He was not pleased with the dramatic increase in triglycerides and questioned me strenuously about my diet. He truly believed I was eating chocolate and other sweets and/or drinking alcohol. Because he did not know about the HeartStopper Effect, he could not see the connection between the increased carbohydrates and drastically reduced fat of the Ornish Diet and my sudden jump in triglycerides. In his paradigm, the Ornish Diet was working, except I was cheating on my diet.

Only after I strenuously objected did he accept that I was not drinking alcohol or gorging on sweets. Before he could crack the mystery, I moved from Des Moines and found a new cardiologist, Dr. Frank Carrea, who, fortunately for me, knew all about the HeartStopper Effect. I was fortunate that a couple of years earlier he had attended a seminar held by Dr. Robert Superko, director of the Lipid Institute. Dr. Superko is a leading researcher in the treatment of small-particle LDL syndrome. He is highly motivated; he has the disease himself.

With the hugely elevated levels of triglycerides and the worsening cholesterol/HDL ratio that my extremely low-fat diet was causing, I suspect my risk factors for developing more dangerous plaque were increasing.

MY BLOOD VALUES WITH 1,000 Mg NIACIN, 20 Mg STATIN (2/6/97)

Total Cholesterol	High Density Lipoproteins (HDL)	Low Density Lipoproteins (LDL)	Triglycerides
178	53	103	114

Cholesterol/HDL ratio = 3.4:1 (average risk)

Look at the dramatic change in my blood values in eight months. Although these changes might not be typical for all heart patients, in my case, by abandoning an extremely low-fat diet and actually *increasing* fat intake, and by taking niacin and a cholesterol-reducing drug, I was suddenly in the normal range of heart attack risk.

Let's examine some of the details in this information. A key ratio is the one between total cholesterol and HDL. The ideal is somewhere around 3:1—for example, a total cholesterol of 180 with an HDL of 60. As the ratio becomes larger in favor of total cholesterol, the greater the heart attack risk over time. My original ratio was about 6:1, a bad ratio. I had at least triple the heart attack risk of a normal male my age from this ratio alone, not even considering the increased risk of my high cholesterol, high LDL, and high triglycerides.

Remember earlier I mentioned how some people could have a high cholesterol level and still not be at risk of a heart attack?

Well, it's because of this ratio. With an HDL level of 90, one could have a total cholesterol level of 270 and be at average risk. Or, with a total cholesterol around 180, this person's ratio would be 2:1. His arteries would probably be clean as a whistle.

However, for someone with a heart-killer gene, a total cholesterol of 180 (normally a great number) coupled with an HDL of 30 would yield a ratio of 6:1, a ticking time bomb. This is why it is so important to have blood tests periodically and to request more than just a simple cholesterol count. Normally, an individual gets just a total cholesterol test. Look at the previous example. The person's cholesterol is 180. Most doctors seeing that would tell you that you are doing well with a cholesterol under 200. Particularly if you are enrolled in an HMO, your doctor would probably not order more specific blood tests because it would seem unnecessary. But unless you do the full lipid panel, you don't know that your total cholesterol level is deceptive. It really is terrible considering the cholesterol/HDL ratio. You need help fast! Yet you leave your doctor's office lulled into the false sense that you are doing just fine.

If you're lucky, you wake up in the middle of the night with a heart attack. If you're not lucky, well, you just won't wake up. If you're really lucky, you find out about the HeartStopper Effect while there is still time to do something about it.

In my case, my cardiologist has the following goals: total cholesterol 150–175; HDL above 45; LDL under 100; triglycerides under 100. These are somewhat aggressive goals. But that's the point; they're goals. If I can stay near them, my body should have converted from its natural state of producing small-particle LDLs (Type B Subpattern) to producing large-particle LDLs (Type A Subpattern). Whatever plaque I have should be stable, not likely to crack or peel, and not growing. I shouldn't be growing clots the size of Cincinnati to block my coronary arteries.

We've all heard about how women are less prone to heart attacks than men. This is because, until menopause, estrogen protects women in three ways. First, estrogen relaxes artery walls and causes lower blood pressure; clots are less likely to form when blood pressure is low. Second, estrogen increases HDL (good cholesterol) production. Third, estrogen decreases LDL (bad cholesterol) production.

If a woman carries a HeartStopper gene, estrogen masks its effects until after menopause. Then her risk level catches up to that of men. One significant danger for a female carrier is that after decades of good cardiac health, she does not anticipate heart problems. Her dietary habits and activity level have been well established. Diet and exercise that carried her through half a century in good health may now be inadequate to forestall the Heart-Stopper Effect.

Debate rages over estrogen replacement therapy for post-menopausal women. Again, the media has framed the issue by sensationalizing the results of a few studies that showed increased cancer risk for women taking estrogen supplements. Consequently, women's attention has become fixated on the cancer risk of estrogen therapy. But for postmenopausal women who do not take estrogen, *the risk of heart attack is three to four times the risk of developing cancer.* To make an informed decision, a woman needs to have information on both cancer and heart attack risks.

Another significant factor in the HeartStopper Effect is smoking. If you smoke, you need to solve that problem first. All the ratios and risks are meaningless if you throw in smoking. Why? Because smoking reduces the body's production of protective HDL and increases the production of damaging LDL. For women, the protective effects of estrogen are neutralized by smoking. This is why in the past twenty years women's heart attack rates have increased correspondingly to the increase in women's smoking rates.

Remember that the HeartStopper gene reduces HDL production and increases LDL production. So, if you smoke, you are assisting in its work. I never smoked and this damnable disease blew away one-third of my heart at age forty-five. If I had smoked, it might have taken me much earlier. I had two male cousins (heavy smokers) whom I suspect had the HeartStopper Effect because both died of heart attacks at an early age: one at forty-three and the other at thirty-five.

Once favorable blood lipid levels are reached, can we relax, throw away the medications, and celebrate? The answer is no. If we stop therapy, our systems will revert to their normal small-particle propensity and will get back to the business of packing cholesterol on our arteries until it kills us.

Therapy is for life (pardon the pun).

CHAPTER 5

The Cadillac Mask

Every morning around five-thirty, I was awakened by the X-ray technician. He would slip a flat plastic box about two feet square behind me, line up the X-ray projector, and zap me. The box contained the film. It was always icy cold when he pushed my naked back against it. It was a wake-up call I dreaded.

I read his name tag. "Steve, do you refrigerate these plates every morning?"

"Just for you."

"Stethoscopes, electrodes, everything that comes in contact with human flesh has to be chilled first? That's the rule?"

"You betcha." Steve wore a lopsided grin.

"I'm glad I don't need a gynecologist."

Without missing a beat, Steve said, "Yeah, those guys dip the speculum in liquid nitrogen just before use."

I laughed so hard I started to cough.

I have incredibly good hearing. It has enabled me all my life to hear conversations that the participants think are private. I caught snatches of conversation in the halls between my doctors and the nurses. On my fifth day in the ICU, I heard my cardiologist tell the charge nurse, "On the X ray, his lungs look like a lake. Watch his oxygen saturation. He acts better than he looks."

I was on pure oxygen and I did have trouble breathing. From the looks I caught from the corner of my eye, I sensed the doctor wasn't telling me how concerned he was. I realized that my family and the staff were keeping things from me. Why do they do that? Why do they think that a patient can't handle the truth? I found out later that my family was worried that shocking news might bring on another heart attack or sap my will to live.

Two days later, I heard my cardiologist in the hall again: "He's starting into pneumonia. I'm hearing some rales when he breathes."

A shiver went through me. Pneumonia scared me more than the heart attack. The idea of slowly choking and drowning to death reminded me of my first waking hours after the heart attack and that damned trachea tube.

I didn't know then that a weak heart lacks the strength to pump the body's other fluids and they begin to settle in the lungs. I had a lung problem that was largely due to the weakened status of my heart.

For five days, doing the same thing over and over had not improved my condition. I was getting worse. At the edge of a cliff, there isn't much room for error. Something had to change. I just didn't know what. I was outwardly calm, but my mind was racing. I did not intend to go down with pneumonia.

My thoughts kept coming back to the oxygen. I had a soft plastic mask over my nose and mouth. It blasted cool, moist air into my face all day and all night. I had dubbed it the Cadillac Mask because it reminded me of driving in a big Cadillac convertible with the top down on a humid summer night. The nurses also began calling it the Cadillac Mask, and I'm told the name stuck after I left.

The oxygen. It seemed to me that the human body was not designed for pure oxygen. And the moisture. If my lungs were filling with water, humidity seemed like the last thing I needed.

I began to experiment by taking off the Cadillac Mask and watching the oxygen monitor. My blood saturation dropped from 98 percent down to the mid eighties. I replaced the mask and it rose. Then I tried holding the mask on my stomach, but allowing the oxygen to blow up into my face. The monitor settled in around 90 percent. The staff wanted my saturation level in the high nineties, but as long as I didn't feel dizzy, I let it drift lower to avoid breathing directly through the mask.

I did this all day, allowing the moist oxygen to blend with the dry, air-conditioned room air. I don't know how I came upon this technique. I just did it. By evening, my blood oxygen level was again in the mid nineties, but I was barely using the mask. My body was readjusting to normal air.

By the time I went to sleep, I had weaned myself off oxygen. Of course, the nurses were not happy with this and wanted me to sleep with the mask on, but I kept pointing to the monitor. "If my blood has a ninety-five percent oxygen saturation, what's the problem?"

"What if you have trouble during the night?"

"Then I'll put the mask back on."

They watched me closely that night, but by morning, my blood oxygen was at 98 percent and the Cadillac Mask was resting on the bed beside me, hissing away at ninety miles an hour. That morning's X ray showed a dramatic improvement in my lungs. They were clearing.

Later that day, my cardiologist asked me what I had done and I explained my weaning technique of the previous day. He asked about what I had discovered and how it had worked for me. He congratulated me on my success. Is this a solution for other patients? I don't know. Maybe my body was ready to heal and my weaning off oxygen was a coincidence. Yet considering my doctor's comments from the halls, I had been getting worse for days.

The nurse, who the previous day had fought with me about taking off my oxygen mask, kept checking my blood oxygen. She could not accept that I was better.

Later that day, one of the ER nurses popped in for a brief chat. She had been on duty the night the ambulance delivered me. She and several other ER nurses kept checking on me every day. I was pleased with this and used every visit as an opportunity to pick their memories to find out what had happened that night.

The nurse admitted the ER staff were amazed I was still alive. She and the others who popped in sporadically would hang around for a few minutes and chat. Then before they left, they'd always touch me. I don't think they were aware of it, but I noted that every one of them did it on each visit. It was as if I were a talisman, a charm, from which they might draw luck or inspiration.

The ICU staff would usually collar these ER visitors in the hall, and I would hear various viewpoints of my story discussed over and over. I felt as if I were an alien phenomenon that had been dropped in their midst, leaving a wake of consternation.

After I got rid of the Cadillac Mask and my pneumonia disappeared, the ICU staff also started calling me Miracle Man.

Outwardly, I took these attentions lightheartedly, another detail to quip about, but inside I knew these were not miracles. I was fighting for my life using the only organ of my body that hadn't been weakened: my brain.

The experience with the Cadillac Mask was my first step in developing my own treatment. As I thought about it, I was disturbed that, although my experimentation with my oxygen supply had yielded a significant result, not only had the medical staff tried to stop me in my oxygen-weaning, but afterward showed little interest in discovering how and why this approach had worked. Though I did not consciously realize at the time that I *had* to become an active force in determining what would be done to me, subconsciously some force was emerging, some instinct was taking over. I was bucking the system.

This was not an easy step. Like most people, I grew up with the myth that doctors were all-knowing creatures who dispensed their wisdom for us lesser mortals and our only option was to obey or suffer. The Doctor Myth is a part of our culture. As with all paradigms, it is difficult to step out of the box of our own thinking.

In the Doctor Myth, the doctor takes on the role of priest or rabbi. He has a special connection to divine wisdom. If one does not obey his edicts, one stays sick or gets sicker. On the other hand, obedience yields a return to health. It's powerful stuff.

Having faced the ultimate consequence, perhaps I was less worried about the much smaller consequences my rebellions might cause. I had seen fate's ultimate surprise, so what could some doctors and nurses possibly do that was worse? The jolting experience of death and rebirth may have rearranged my thinking. Whatever the reasons, somewhere inside me there was a voice, a new part of me, that began to question everything. In those first days in the hospital, I was not aware of this voice, but it was gently tugging me toward an approach to medicine that was very different from the rules of the Doctor Myth I had known all my life.

In the Doctor Myth, the doctor makes the decisions; the patient obeys. But I was beginning to view treatment of my disease very differently. In my developing idea, the experts in technique, the doctors and nurses, provided expert analysis to the patient, who then weighed alternatives. Using a sports analogy, it's easy to put the doctor in the role of quarterback, but the patient must be the leader. The players must all work together, each bringing skills to the game, and being led by a patient-quarterback who makes the calls. Information may come from the other team members, but it is the patient's life on the line.

I truly believe that many medical malpractice lawsuits result from patient ignorance, from having total faith that the doctor knows everything and will fix all the patient's problems. When this doesn't happen, when the heightened expectations are not met, then the patient is disappointed and angry. Unfortunately, when less than perfection is achieved in curing the patient's disease, the lawyers are called in to punish the doctor.

Granted, some malpractice lawsuits are the result of doctors' mistakes; others are the result of greed. But many are filed by angry patients who did not get the results they expected. Unfortunately, the Doctor Myth fosters a belief in magic. The patient's part in the magical deal is to obey and believe; the doctor's part is to concoct some medication or perform some procedure to solve the patient's problem. But if a patient does not understand the problem, he or she can't possibly understand the probabilities of a specific outcome. No specific outcome is ever certain.

It amazes me that people will shop around for an auto mechanic, bedevil the poor bugger with a thousand questions about what he intends to do to their car, and then haggle over a $10 part. But when it comes to their lives, people are largely willing to lie back, nod their head, and let a doctor make decisions that will have far more impact on them than a new clutch.

In the hospital I watched entire families sit in silence as doctors told them what was wrong with their relatives and how they intended to treat the ailments. Only after the doctors departed did these families talk amongst themselves, raising questions and concerns that none of them could answer. Perhaps seeing that triggered in me the realization that I had to interrogate the doctors and nurses. I needed to squeeze from them everything they knew if I was to have a chance of survival. And if I failed, then at least my life had been in my hands.

CHAPTER 6

Detecting
the HeartStopper Effect

Without blood tests, without fancy diagnostics, you can determine how likely you are to have a heart attack by looking at your relatives. As I have learned, one of the most significant early indicators is your family's cardiac history. Half the people who have heart disease have a first-degree relative with heart disease.

Since the HeartStopper Effect is an inherited disease, someone else in your bloodline had to pass it to you. Have direct blood relatives, particularly parents or grandparents, had heart attacks? Were they younger than fifty when they did? An affirmative answer to both of these questions is a strong indicator of possible HeartStopper heredity.

Have direct blood relatives had strokes? The unstable plaque that causes blood clots that trigger a heart attack can also form clots that go to the brain and cause strokes.

Do you or direct blood relatives have high blood pressure? Though high blood pressure is not a direct effect of a killer gene, having high blood pressure increases your risk of blood clots. Remember how unstable plaque can trigger an artery-blocking clot? The likelihood of a killer clot is increased by high blood pressure, so managing blood pressure is very important if you have a killer gene.

If you answered yes to more than two of the above questions, you are at higher than normal risk for heart attack or stroke. What should you do now?

Having a blood lipid panel done is a good first step in detecting heart disease. This test is routine and should be covered by most health insurance plans. It costs around $20 to $30. Who should have this blood test? I believe that every adult, regardless of family history, should have a complete blood workup to assess general health and to establish a base of data to measure against in the future. Sometime after the early twenties, say about twenty-five, would be a good time to start assessing one's blood lipids. Doctors don't feel blood tests are very revealing for children, unless there is a strong hereditary line of heart attacks in a child's family. Heart disease builds up over time, so the sooner one knows of its existence, the sooner one can begin making changes to forestall disaster.

After you get the results of your lipid panel, what should you look for? The next chart shows you the values your blood should have. (Note: all readings in milligrams/deciliter of blood [mg/dL]. The symbol ≤ means less than or equal to; ≥ means greater than or equal to.)

HEALTHY TARGET BLOOD VALUES

Total Cholesterol	High Density Lipoproteins (HDL)	Low Density Lipoproteins (LDL)	Triglycerides
High: ≥ 250 Desired: ≤ 200	Low: ≤ 40 Desired: Men ≥ 45 Women ≥ 55	High: ≥ 160 Desired: ≤ 130	High: ≥ 250 Desired: ≤ 140

The scores in the chart above can be used as targets by anyone. Those who have a heart-killer gene or who have experienced coronary blockage or a heart attack may want to be more aggressive, such as I've been in my own personal goals, shown in this next chart.

AGGRESSIVE TARGET BLOOD VALUES

Total Cholesterol	High Density Lipoproteins (HDL)	Low Density Lipoproteins (LDL)	Triglycerides
Ideal: ≤ 180	Ideal: ≥ 45	Ideal: ≤ 100	Ideal: ≤ 100

So how do your test scores compare? If they are within the limits I've outlined, your arteries should be in great shape. However, be warned that some individuals may have excellent lipid panel results and still exhibit the HeartStopper Effect.

If your results are way outside the above values, does this mean you have a heart-killer gene? Not necessarily. Look further.

Divide your total cholesterol score by your HDL score. This produces your cholesterol/HDL ratio, an important indicator. If the number that results is less than 4:1, you have what is considered to be a healthy ratio. If it is between 4:1 and 5:1, doctors recommend that you should try some short-term remedies such as more exercise, diet control, weight loss, etc., under the guidance of your doctor. If your ratio is over 5:1, you have double or triple the likelihood of a heart attack compared to the general population, though it may not be caused by a HeartStopper gene.

The next chart shows the relative risks of various cholesterol/HDL ratios.

CHOLESTEROL/HDL RATIOS

≤ 3:1 Low Risk	3:1 to 4:1 Average Risk	4.1:1 to 6:1 2X Risk	6.1:1 to 8:1 3X Risk	8.1:1 to 10:1 4X Risk	≥ 10:1 Extreme Risk

The lipid panel can only suggest that you have potential heart disease; it does not identify the specific cause. If your blood values are out of the desired ranges and your cholesterol/HDL ratio is risky, if you're overweight and eat junk food, the chances are large that you have run-of-the-mill coronary artery disease. So, the next step is to rule this out. I suggest you begin to exercise regularly, shift your diet away from fats and sweets, and start losing weight. If you lose weight, then in two to three months have another lipid panel done. If your blood levels and ratio move into or closer to the optimum ranges shown in the charts, then you have solved your problem and probably don't have a genetic component. However, if your blood values and your cholesterol/HDL ratio haven't changed much, you may have a killer gene, because even moderate exercise and weight loss should otherwise have a fairly dramatic effect on your numbers. The next step is to have the specific blood test that identifies the HeartStopper Effect.

Let's review and quantify the potential risks. Inherited familial hyperlipidemia, with high LDL and high triglycerides, increases the risk of coronary events fourfold. If the LDL being produced is small-particle, this increases the risk another threefold. A total-cholesterol-to-HDL ratio of more than 4:1 doubles cardiac risk. As you can see, the typical manifestation of a killer gene—low HDL, high triglycerides, and high LDL—typically gives one a coronary risk *nine times* that of a normal person. And this is a generality. Depending on one's habits, this risk can be even higher. If one eats fatty foods, drinks alcohol heavily, smokes, and is a couch potato, the risk can be much higher.

What if you're not a couch potato? If you are already athletic, in the normal weight range for your height, and eat a highly nutritious diet, and your first lipid panel shows blood values in the danger zones, then you have a high probability of carrying a killer gene. It's ironic that the people who look healthiest and who are the least likely to suspect coronary problems are exactly those who are most vulnerable because they are not looking for heart disease symptoms; they think they're healthy. If you already live a healthy lifestyle and your bloodwork has values in the danger zones, there is no reason to wait two or three months to see if these values will come down. You should immediately be tested for the presence of abundant small-particle LDL, the HeartStopper Effect.

For this test, which is called *gradient gel electrophoresis,* a small sample of blood is drawn and analyzed for its content of small-particle LDL as well as for specific protein markers of various killer genes. This test is considered conclusive.

Your doctor can have your LDL subclass tested in one of two ways. First is to find a nearby university hospital or research facility to perform gradient gel electrophoresis. This is not easy because these facilities usually provide testing services only for their own researchers and staff. The other alternative is to use the one commercial lab that will perform the test for any doctor in the country. Here's the address:

Detecting the HeartStopper Effect

Berkeley HeartLab, Inc.
1311 Harbor Bay Parkway, Suite 1004
Alameda, CA 94502
800-432-7889

Your doctor will need to order a test kit that contains the proper sample containers and reagents from Berkeley HeartLab, Inc. You take the kit to a local blood laboratory, where a blood sample will be drawn and packaged into the special kit, which will be sent by overnight courier to the testing lab. In a couple of weeks, your doctor should receive the test results and an analysis of your results. These tests determine the existence of apolipoprotein B, apolipoprotein E and its subclasses, lipoprotein (a), as well as other genetic markers for heart disease. Most important, the tests identify levels of small, dense LDL particles, the markers for the HeartStopper Effect.

Some local blood labs test for apolipoprotein B, apolipoprotein E and its subclasses, and lipoprotein (a), but they cannot determine small-particle LDL levels. You could be tested for the presence of one of these gene mutations to help narrow down whether you might have a propensity for the HeartStopper Effect, but you won't know for sure until your blood goes through the gradient gel electrophoresis test. This is a sensitive test, developed by the National Institutes of Health, that requires expensive equipment and constant recalibration and monitoring for accuracy. High start-up cost is one reason the testing is not widely available from local labs. There's also a big catch-22. Since most doctors don't know about the HeartStopper Effect, there is no demand for labs to test for LDL subclasses; since commercial labs don't provide the testing nationwide, doctors can't ask for it.

Several gene mutations can cause the HeartStopper Effect. More will probably be discovered. The exact mechanisms by which each of these genes upsets the body's fat management are not fully known. However, if a gene causes the final effect of high small-particle LDL production, treatment is possible.

If you are significantly overweight, you might want to ask your doctor to request the test for the existence of apolipoproteins E1,

2, 3, and 4. ApoE4, in particular, manifests itself in obesity and dangerously high total-cholesterol levels: 300, 400, and higher. Some patients have total cholesterol counts over 1,000. For these patients, cholesterol-reducing drugs are essential. Some patients don't want to take this test because the existence of the ApoE4 gene is also a high-risk marker for development of Alzheimer's disease. Having this test is a choice only you can make. Recognize that your doctor must tell you about the Alzheimer's risk (49 to 99 percent) before ordering the test and will not conduct the test unless you are willing to be notified if the result shows you have the ApoE4 gene. If you don't want to know that you're at high risk to develop Alzheimer's disease, your doctor probably won't administer the test.

Most health plans cover bloodwork, even genetic tests. A lipid panel is not an expensive test ($20–$30). The screening for small-particle LDL costs around $250. Even if your health plan does not cover it, this test is crucial if your lipid panel shows values significantly beyond the thresholds I have shown in the charts above, or if you have a strong family history of heart disease.

After you have had a lipid panel, if you request the test for LDL small-particle syndrome, you may get some resistance from your doctor, especially if he or she is a general practitioner. One reason is that cholesterol levels (total, HDL, and LDL) are not flagged as dangerous by most laboratories until they are generally higher that the levels I have recommended. So, on your local lab report, there may be no asterisks next to your blood values because the lab does not consider them abnormal. Recognize that your doctor was educated at least five, ten, maybe thirty years ago. Only recently have cholesterol subcomponents become important in diagnosing heart disease. And only in the past few years has diagnosis included the sub-subfractions of cholesterol (such as small, dense LDL particles) with their devastating impact on coronary arteries. Your doctor may not be up-to-date on this material.

A HeartStopper gene is a subtle killer: it does not necessarily create the grossly obvious blood levels that would catch the average general practitioner's diagnostic eye. One's blood levels may not look that far from normal, as in my case. That is why you must get past a doctor's possible resistance and get more advanced bloodwork if your lipid panel shows a cholesterol/HDL ratio over 5:1; HDL under 45 for men or 55 for women; and LDL pushing above 140. Particularly if you have a history of heart attacks in your family, you owe it to yourself to get the conclusive data that an LDL small-particle screening will provide.

The reliance on a lipid panel as the gold standard of cardiac diagnosis has limitations: only patients with "high" total cholesterol, LDL, and triglyceride levels are treated for heart disease. Patients with "normal" test results slip through the diagnostic net unless they complain of chest pain or dizziness. Could this be why half the people who have heart attacks have had no prior warning that they have heart disease?

Doctors unfamiliar with LDL subclasses can make a big diagnostic mistake when dealing with small-particle LDL. If you have high total cholesterol and high LDL, doctors commonly prescribe a cholesterol-lowering statin. These drugs should lower your total cholesterol and LDL. Thus, your doctor thinks he's reversed your march toward coronary artery disease and heart attack. Nothing could be further from the truth. If you are among the 50 percent of coronary artery disease patients who have an LDL subclass disorder, cholesterol-reducing drugs may lower your LDL, *but they don't alter the characteristics of that LDL.* In other words, if your LDL is composed of a high proportion of small, dense particles—the hallmark of the HeartStopper Effect— cholesterol-reducing drugs won't change this proportion. You're still at risk, but you think you're doing great because your lipid panel shows that your LDL level has dropped. This is another danger of relying too heavily on the lipid panel as a diagnostic.

If you still think *your* doctor is an infallible god, consider this. In 1996, Dr. Robert Superko, of the Cholesterol Research Center at the University of California at Berkeley, conducted a study to test the accuracy of the diagnostic assumptions doctors use to interpret lipid panels. In this study, the lipid panel results of 405 patients were used. Using generally accepted assumptions of what constituted low, normal, and high cholesterol, HDL, LDL, and triglycerides, Dr. Superko used patient test results to make predictions about which patients were LDL subclass Type A and which were Type B. Then the gradient gel electrophoresis test was performed for each patient.

The study assumed that triglycerides between 90 and 139 mg/dL were normal and that patients having this triglyceride range would be LDL subclass Pattern A (normal). The predictions were wrong 42 percent of the time.

The study also assumed that triglycerides between 140 and 180 mg/dL were high and would indicate LDL subclass Pattern B (abnormal). The predictions were wrong 21 percent of the time.

Because high HDL is considered beneficial, the study assumed that a fairly high HDL, between 41 and 55 mg/dL, would signal Pattern A for LDL subclass. These predictions were wrong 50 percent of the time.

How acceptable do you think an error rate between 21 and 50 percent is when the doctor is making life-and-death decisions about your health?

Consider that you may be among the carriers who do not manifest abnormal lipid panel results. My suggestion is that if you have direct blood relatives (especially if more than one) who have had heart attacks, you should skip lipid panels and get the LDL subclass test. Since 50 percent of heart disease patients have first-degree relatives with heart disease, and since 80 percent of coronary artery disease patients do not have abnormal lipid panels, you could have the HeartStopper Effect and have no indication detectable by regular testing.

If your bloodwork is significantly outside the norms in the above charts or if you have definite hereditary risk, be persistent. Have your doctor call Dr. Robert Superko at Berkeley HeartLab, Inc., and get brought up to speed on this disease. Lend your doctor my book. Or if your doctor is adamant, get a second opinion. If all else fails, pay for the test yourself.

Unless you like sleepless nights.

Finding out you have the HeartStopper Effect is not the end of the world. The end of the world is not knowing you have it. In fact, if you have not yet had a heart attack, it's time for celebration. The stealth killer didn't creep up on you fast enough; now that you know it's there, you can combat it.

Treatment is not difficult, particularly if you catch the condition before having a heart attack. First, make sure you see a cardiologist. You need expert advice. Then, begin a regimen of exercise, diet, and stress reduction. Most important, you need to start taking medications.

Here's one catch. Many doctors, including cardiologists, do not know about this genetic condition. It has not been widely publicized. Some doctors may resist your suggestions of a genetic problem. Stick to your guns and insist on a small-particle LDL screening. If your doctor pooh-poohs your suggestions and wants to treat you as a run-of-the-mill patient who wants to lower cholesterol, maybe you should look for another doctor. The treatment for the killer gene's effect—small-particle LDL syndrome—is *different* from other cholesterol-reduction and weight-reduction treatments. But if your doctor tries to lower your cholesterol through traditional treatments—primarily a low-fat diet—he or she could do you harm.

Over the past few years, numerous articles have appeared about a condition the media has named Syndrome X. The more descriptive clinical name of this disease is insulin resistance.

The effects of Syndrome X and a HeartStopper gene are similar: both can create high cholesterol, high LDL, high triglycerides, bad total-cholesterol/HDL ratios, and high risk of heart attack. But they are not the same.

Syndrome X may have a different genetic cause. Syndrome X manifests itself in the body's inability to get glucose into body cells.

The human digestive system is designed to break down food into simple components of sugar (glucose) and fat (lipoproteins). The bloodstream then delivers these simple sugars and fats to all cells in the body for use in the production of energy, cell repair, and growth. In a normal body, when a glucose molecule approaches a cell, receptors in the cell's surface are triggered by insulin in the bloodstream. These receptors recognize the glucose and let it through the cell membrane. The body produces insulin to regulate the use of glucose in its cells: when it wants more glucose to be absorbed, it produces more insulin to tell the cells to accept glucose; when it wants to dampen glucose absorption, it produces less insulin. In people with Syndrome X, this process is hampered: cells don't readily let glucose enter. The body then produces more and more insulin to force the cells to accept glucose. The result of all this is high glucose levels in the bloodstream, which stimulates the liver to produce cholesterol. In extreme cases, the patient becomes diabetic.

People afflicted with insulin resistance are usually overweight and sometimes grossly obese; they do not exercise; they frequently have high sugar and fat intakes. Treatment for Syndrome X is fairly simple: exercise and adopting a healthy diet with drastic reductions in sugar and fat. By following this regimen, patients lose weight, their blood sugar levels drop, their cholesterol levels move into the normal range, and the cells of their body are no longer insulin resistant.

In contrast, carriers of a HeartStopper gene are not necessarily overweight. They may already exercise and have what are normally considered healthy diets. Though exercise and a healthy diet are helpful, by themselves they will not counter the Heart-Stopper Effect.

If you are a couch potato who has recently been alarmed by a high cholesterol count, a good way to tell the difference between Syndrome X and the effects of a HeartStopper gene would be to start exercising and adopting a healthy diet. If you begin to lose weight and your cholesterol level drops after a few months, then chances are you do not have a HeartStopper gene. If you started with a bad cholesterol/HDL ratio and it moves into the normal range (3:1 to 4:1), you probably do not have a HeartStopper gene.

Another clue doctors use to distinguish between these two killers is blood glucose levels. A HeartStopper gene does not seem to affect glucose usage, while Syndrome X causes high blood glucose levels. When you look at the results of your blood tests, check the glucose level. If your level is high (above 100) and you have high cholesterol and triglycerides, you should probably first determine if you have insulin resistance before assuming you have a HeartStopper gene. (You may be diabetic or prediabetic.) Before drawing conclusions, you need to lose weight and exercise as explained above. However, if your blood glucose level is below 100, you probably don't have Syndrome X.

Though the effects of Syndrome X are serious, they are easily reversed and don't usually require medication. However, to reverse the effects of a HeartStopper gene, you must at the very least start niacin therapy to increase your HDL level. In more critical cases such as mine, it may also be necessary to take a cholesterol-reducing drug.

If you have high blood pressure, weight control is essential. In more severe cases, you may need to take a medication to keep blood pressure under control. Daily aspirin therapy is also a good idea to lessen the clotting potential caused by unstable plaque. If you have unstable plaque, you want to reduce it or turn it into stable plaque to reduce your danger of a sudden, artery-blocking clot. Because aspirin reduces blood's ability to clot, it offers powerful protection against the mechanism that actually triggers a heart attack. One aspirin a day can cut the incidence of heart attack by almost 50 percent.

Research activity on HeartStopper genes is still so small, there is no conclusive evidence on exactly how they work. The most current theory involves the interaction of LDL receptors in the liver with LDL levels in the blood. As an analogy, consider your stomach. When you eat a meal, receptors in the stomach signal the brain that the stomach is full. The brain then informs you to stop gathering food (well, except at Thanksgiving, when this mechanism seems not to work). You stop eating until stomach receptors later tell your brain the stomach is empty and you are "hungry." This is called a feedback loop.

In the case of fat levels in the blood, LDL receptors in the liver sense when LDL levels exceed normal. These receptors then inform the rest of the liver to slow down LDL production. When the LDL level drops below normal, the same receptors signal the liver to produce more LDL. It is theorized that a killer gene affects LDL receptors. Either the afflicted person's LDL receptors are impaired in their ability to sense LDL or there are fewer of the receptors. So, as LDL levels rise, the receptors do not provide the negative feedback to tell the liver to cut LDL production. Not until LDL levels are very high do the impaired receptors perceive sufficient presence of LDL to tell the liver to cut LDL production. "Normal" for a carrier of a HeartStopper gene is really quite abnormal.

These receptors may also be the reason HDL levels are abnormally low in carriers of the gene. If LDL is perceived to be too low, the liver would not produce HDL, which acts as an agent to further reduce LDL.

Since killer genes are a fairly new discovery, researchers still have a long way to go to understand their mechanisms of destruction. However, even though the detailed chemical and molecular functions of these genes are not yet fully understood, enough is known of the gross effects for doctors to treat the condition. Perhaps in the future, simpler, more direct treatments will be discovered, but for the present, we know that niacin and cholesterol-lowering drugs along with diet and exercise are key components of successfully managing this deadly affliction.

And there's some good news. People with Type B LDL subclass (abnormal) respond better to treatment than do Type A (normal) people with normal coronary artery disease.

CHAPTER 7

Secrets

I had a big surprise the first time I was able to get out of bed and use the bathroom. I found it in the bathroom mirror. When I looked at myself, I was almost jolted into another heart attack. My face was puffed up, red, black-and-blue. My eyes were swelling out of their sockets and streaked with bloodshot vessels. None of the whites of my eyes were white. With my hair sticking up in a thousand points of fright, I looked like a monster from a 1950s, grade-B horror movie. I was too hideous to look at. I averted my face from the mirror. I thought of the way Lon Chaney had recoiled from his reflection when he first saw himself turn into a werewolf.

I was stricken when I returned to my bed. I looked at Beverly and was amazed that she would look me in the eyes. I said, "Why didn't you tell me?"

"Honey, you had enough to deal with."

I found that Beverly, my mother, and my brother had agreed not to reveal to me the state of my face. They had taken the hand mirrors out of the hospital room and had not shown me the pop-up mirror in the bedside table. They had also persuaded the doctors and nurses not to talk to me about my face. I was amazed that this conspiracy of silence had held for almost a week.

Once I knew the "ugly" truth, I began asking how it had happened. I heard a slew of conflicting stories. My cardiologist said that during seizures, blood vessels in the eyes and face often rupture, particularly if the patient is on heparin, a blood thinner, as I had been. One of the nurses said she thought I had banged my head against the handrails on the sides of the ER bed when I was thrashing around in seizure. One of the orderlies said he had heard that after I passed out, I had been left in a hallway and had fallen out of the ER bed. He said I was found on the floor in a pool of vomit. To this day, I do not know what actually happened.

It took months for the bruises to disappear. I looked like either a raccoon or a Transylvanian prince. Long after I was mobile and feeling fit, I still had the dark shadows of my ordeal painted across my face. I took to wearing sunglasses whenever I left the house.

I found that my family withheld other information from me as well. A few weeks before my heart attack, I had shipped off my first novel to a literary agent in New York, seeking representation for it. I was sure I had written a best-seller and had been waiting avidly for a response. Every day, I asked family members if the mail had brought word of my manuscript. They always said no.

Not until I got home after two weeks in the hospital did I find that the manuscript had been returned with a rejection letter. Though disappointed, I was not depressed by this. I knew there were thousands of agents and it was only a matter of time before I found one to represent me. I could have handled the news. I was not happy about being kept in the dark.

I can understand my family's concern for keeping unpleasant news from me, but they didn't understand that, having stood on the boundary between life and death, I had drastically altered what I perceived as significant and insignificant. If something was related to my immediate family, it was significant. By contrast, the success or failure of my book, global warming, and nuclear winter were now only small blips on the radar screen of my thoughts.

Only recently, while poring through my hospital records, I was staggered by the notes I found. I uncovered another secret. The notes reveal that during those first days after my heart attack, I was not in danger of going into congestive heart failure, I was *already in* congestive heart failure. My heart was so weak it was not able to move all the necessary fluids through my body. This was why my lungs looked like a "lake" in the X rays. Neither my family nor I had been told how close to the end I was, but one of the doctors had clearly written in my notes that my condition was "grave" and that I "could go at any moment."

As I look back, part of me thinks that maybe I didn't really need to know that secret. I'm sure the doctors felt that telling me I was in congestive heart failure might have sapped my will to live. Perhaps. But I think I should have been told.

The doctors kept certain things from my family, my family kept certain things from me. It's more of the Doctor Myth, information as power. The one in the more powerful position deems when it is appropriate to reveal powerful information, and how much. When you are lying in a hospital bed with tubes inserted and wires attached to you, the feeling of helplessness is probably the greatest it will ever be, no matter who you are. Your job title, your contacts, are meaningless behind the closed doors of the temples of medicine.

Regardless of the feeling of imprisonment, the one thing that is unshackled is your mind. It can roam anywhere, do anything. I trust my mind to deal with what I learn. I want to know what goes on around me. I'll deal with the consequences.

This experience has made me unflinching about the facts of my health. Nothing anyone can tell me will discourage me to the point of giving up. I *chose* to come back here. When my heart can't function anymore, this life will end, but I know where I'm going. Yes, there are unknowns. Yes, they are scary, but I've had the dress rehearsal.

The problem is that my family has not had the experience I've had. They *say* they will not keep information from me in the future, but I wonder if they will be able to give me bad news. I wonder if at crunch time they will worry about the effects and try to protect me rather than letting the one who has to experience the outcome deal with it.

Friends and coworkers frequently ask how facing death has changed me. It's not something I can easily explain and I stumble for an answer. They seem to want me to reveal some profound secret. I get the impression they think I am hoarding valuable information and that I'm unwilling to share.

When I was in the hospital right after my heart attack, I had endless hours to think. I asked myself, "What do you feel right now? Why do you feel it?" I kept trying to assess how I was different. I asked myself, "Would you trade all your money and possessions to walk out of here undamaged right now?"

"Yes."

"What is most important to you?"

"The three people in this room: my fiancée, my mother, and my brother."

As I lay there, locked in my internal dialogue, random images, moments, jumped out of time. I wanted to be sitting on my back porch with the breeze wafting through my hair, the sun in my face, and watching my dog chase a stick across the emerald grass. I wanted to be back on the elevator in San Francisco where I first saw Beverly and then took everyone on the elevator to dinner so I could meet her. I wanted to be in the middle of those seemingly endless summer vacations in our rowboat with my brother catching painted turtles. I wanted to be entering the public library for the first time with my mother, feeling that the size of the world had just tripled as we crossed the threshold hand in hand.

How do you tell people about the importance of the simple moments in your life? How do you explain that no profundities leap into your head when you hover at the edge of infinity? Just the simple moments that you didn't even notice at the time. They are what count because in them there is truth. The rest is stage dressing.

CHAPTER 8

Genetics

In 1994, Time/CNN conducted a survey in which they asked adults if they were interested in taking a genetics test that would tell them what diseases they might expect to get later in life. The results were startling. Fifty percent of those surveyed wanted to know if they had a genetic disease. Forty-nine percent *did not want to know!* This amazes me. Had I known years ago that I carried a HeartStopper gene, I would have done anything to avoid my heart attack.

Over four thousand diseases have been linked to genetic causes. Everything from cancer to heart disease to obesity has genetic linkages. Understanding this changes the way one looks at medicine. For centuries, medicine has focused on treating symptoms. Only now are we able to begin treating the actual causes of disease. Prevention before a disease takes hold is far more powerful than any medical procedure after it has wreaked its damage.

Having a genetically caused disease does not mean one is destined to succumb to it. Many genetically caused diseases are treatable. The HeartStopper Effect can be counteracted by something as simple as taking daily doses of aspirin and niacin, which together cost less than fifty cents per day. Three years ago if someone had explained to me that I had the HeartStopper Effect and had offered me a brochure on how I could prevent my impending near-fatal heart attack for $200 a year, I would have grabbed the brochure so fast the vacuum would have sucked his arm out of its socket.

The psychological aspects of having a genetically caused disease can have an impact on family dynamics. Once a disease is identified in a family, family members start to worry. Members can experience depression, anger, or denial. Fear is also a factor. Even though testing for the HeartStopper Effect requires only a simple blood draw, the anxiety one experiences while waiting for test results can be profound. Even after finding they are not carriers of a specific disease, some family members continue to be fearful. "What if the test was wrong? What if I get it anyway?"

Those who find they carry the disease gene may wish they had never submitted to screening. They may be angry at the other family member(s) who persuaded them to get tested. They may reject treatment. It is difficult to accept that one houses something lethal in one's body, something that won't go away. It is as if one's body has become an enemy. We have no control over such facts, but we resent the assaults on our self-image. It's easy to kill the messenger. Children may resent the parent who gave them the gene. In contrast, those family members who find they do not carry the disease gene may feel guilt that they were spared while other family members will pay the price.

Genetics counselors can help families deal with the shifting dynamics that occur as members discover their carrier status.

I don't like to dwell on what might have been had I known more about my cardiac status before my heart attack. I've gone through the recriminations and the anger and the looking for a scapegoat. No matter what I think, I now have a damaged heart. Nothing will change this. In the end, I have accepted that looking back is fruitless, self-defeating.

I am physically functional at almost my pre-heart-attack level. I can go about my days and enjoy life with minor accommodation of my heart. Yes, I get dizzy if I stand up too fast. Yes, I need frequent naps. Yes, I may feel faint in a hot shower. Yes, I avoid being alone in case something untoward happens. But it is far more important for me to do the things I enjoy and to look to the future than to wallow in the past. I have a direct effect on what will happen to me. I control my exercise, my medication. I would much rather focus on feeling good and helping others avoid heart attacks than regret the years my life has been cut short.

*   *   *

The killer genes are Mendelian dominant genes. This means they are inherited in the classic inheritance scheme discovered by Gregor Mendel in the 1800s. Each gene in the human body comes in pairs; each parent contributes one-half of each pair. Since each parent's genes are also in pairs, there is a 50 percent chance that either of the parents' gene pair components will go to a specific child. "Dominant" means that if either parent gives the child the gene, the gene pair that results will act as if both sides of the gene pair carried the disease. In this case, the child will manifest the disease.

In a simple Mendel chart, we represent the genetic makeups of two parents whose genes are combined to create a child. The two halves of each parent's gene pair (known as alleles) for a particular trait are shown across the side and top of the chart or "Mendel box." Below, we see the four possible combinations of the parents' alleles combined into new gene pairs for offspring. These represent the possible combinations for each child the couple produces. Children's potential gene pairs are shown in the gray boxes.

Mother		O	O
Father	**K**	KO	KO
	O	OO	OO

In the above chart, the father is a carrier of a killer gene in one allele, represented by K, and a noncarrier in the other allele, represented by O. The mother is not a carrier. Depending on which half of the parents' genes combine, there are four different combinations of gene pairs. In any box where a K appears in the child's gene pairs, the child will exhibit the effects of the killer gene.

So we see the following possible combinations: KO, KO, OO, OO. In this case, the parents have a 50 percent chance of producing a child who has a killer gene and who may then pass it on.

What if both parents are partial carriers?

Mother		K	O
	K	KK	KO
Father			
	O	KO	OO

The result is KK, KO, KO, OO. In this case each child has a 75 percent chance of inheriting a killer gene. Recent research also suggests that the child with the genotype KK may manifest more severe effects of a HeartStopper gene: higher LDL cholesterol levels, more small-particle LDL, lower HDL.

What if one of the parents got the gene from both grandparents so that he has the double gene KK?

Mother		O	O
	K	KO	KO
Father			
	K	KO	KO

In this case, *all* children of this couple will carry and show the effects of the killer gene.

The inevitable question for a carrier of a killer gene is whether to have children. This, of course, is a personal choice. My opinion is that having knowledge of the gene would put the parents in a good position to teach their child good nutrition at an early age. It would mean making sure that blood levels were periodically checked. As the child entered adulthood, it would probably mean the start of drug therapy, either with a cholesterol-lowering drug or niacin, or both, depending on the severity of the symptoms. The objective would be to prevent the crossover to small-particle LDL production in order to prevent plaque buildup.

How difficult would this be? Imagine fighting the effects of TV commercials not merely to prevent tooth decay, but to save a child's life.

If the parents of this theoretical child had begun adopting the dietary habits necessary to thwart the effects of their own killer genes, the child would learn from an early age what foods to eat and what foods not to eat. The food rituals that the parents might have had such a difficult time reversing would not exist in the child. The parents would have the opportunity to create food habits and rituals that the child would find normal.

How many times have we seen children turn their noses up at some food because they have never had it before? If you never feed a child a cheeseburger, will he reject it if offered? Will it become the equivalent of broccoli?

Maybe this is my fantasy, but I believe parents can successfully affect the early food habits of their children. This means going against the prevailing reinforcement behaviors parents themselves learned in which sugar plays a major role in celebration and reward. For instance, instead of rewarding a child with candy, Dad could give the child a pony ride on his back or do something else the child finds enjoyable. Rewards do not always have to be food. A clean room or good grades could be rewarded with a trip to the movies. Birthday cake may be unavoidable, but many other food traditions can be replaced with nonfood pleasures.

Small children cry and get upset, and sugar is effective in

calming them down and getting desired behaviors. But if you have the HeartStopper Effect, think of what you are setting your child up for in the future.

Your food habits and your example have a strong effect on small children. As children approach adulthood and can be taught about the processes in their bodies, example can give way to education.

A child who inherits the HeartStopper Effect will have to be under a doctor's care for the rest of his life, but with a well-balanced diet, exercise, and drug therapy, this child can live out a normal life span.

Once I found out that my killer gene was a Mendelian dominant gene, I immediately began working on my brother to have a lipid panel done on his blood. I knew he had at least a fifty-fifty chance of having the same gene. Since he is only four years younger than me, I thought he might not have much time left.

Despite having seen me almost dead, my brother resisted. He did not want to believe he had this gene. The best I could get from him was that he intended to step up his exercise, cut his fat consumption, and lose weight. Unlike me, he had been border-line hypertensive. Not good.

He dropped about fifteen pounds over the next three months. Then, when he thought he was in great shape, he went to a doctor and had a blood lipid panel done. He expected good results as a reward for his hard work. He was shocked at the report of his bloodwork. His blood levels shattered his self-image. His cholesterol and triglycerides were both near 300. His LDL was near 200. His HDL was low. His blood levels were worse than mine had been before I had my heart attack. His risk of a heart attack was enormous.

It looked very much as if he had a killer gene. He immediately wanted to have the LDL subclass test. Suddenly he was motivated. Sure enough, his results showed he had exactly the same killer gene, the ApoB, I had. We had both inherited our father's fatal flaw. My brother is now on niacin therapy and his blood levels look very good. With luck, he'll not have a heart attack.

Why was he so difficult to convince? Maybe for the same

reason that change is difficult for most people. We each have a body image: we think of ourselves as healthy even if we are overweight or smoke or drink. When someone suggests something might be wrong inside us, we resist this idea because it threatens the self-image we have. It is not easy to think of some disease growing inside one's body. Only after great soul-searching are we able to readjust our perceptions of who we really are.

Even though I can feel the effects of my heart attack—less stamina, sensitivity to cold, occasional faintness—I still find myself believing it never happened. I want to forget I have a damaged heart. Somehow it makes me feel like less than I was. So, if I sometimes have trouble accepting this reality, I can understand how people with no outward signs of the disease would have even more difficulty realigning their thinking.

But consider this. Numerous studies have been done on the risk of coronary artery disease in direct relatives (parents, children, and siblings). They show that a family history of heart disease increases an individual's risk of having a heart attack by at least two to five times normal. Having first-degree relatives who have had coronary artery disease or heart attacks is the most significant factor in determining how likely you are to develop heart disease. It pays to research the health histories of grandparents, aunts, and uncles. Knowing your genetic history can save your life.

I was flabbergasted. Out of nowhere, someone contacted me to see if we were related because we shared the same last name. After trading E-mails with this fellow, he called me. We exchanged stories and I found that his grandfather was my grandfather's brother. I had vague childhood memories of his father, but the two branches of our families could have been on separate planets all these years.

My distant cousin seemed thrilled to have found a long-lost family member in his first week of owning a computer. I, of course, self-absorbed in all things cardiac, asked him about the health of his parents, siblings, and other relatives. What quickly emerged was a story of devastation. His grandfather and granduncle had died of heart attacks in their early fifties. (Memories are dim on exact facts.) His father died of a heart attack at forty-three; his father's brother at thirty-five. Several aunts in his branch of the family had high cholesterol, high blood pressure.

Without thinking, I blurted out that the Bayan line was plagued by a killer gene. I told him of my father's death at fifty, my grandfather's at fifty-seven, then of my close brush with death. I couldn't see his face, but I suspected it was ashen. He was thirty-two and said he had occasional chest pain and that his cholesterol was high. He was scared after I told him that every male, along with several females, on both sides of our family must have had the HeartStopper Effect.

I reassured him that the gene was treatable, but he was concerned because his wife was two months pregnant. Would his child inherit the curse?

I was numb. With each child having a fifty-fifty chance of inheriting the killer gene, what were the odds that every male in three generations would lose this lottery?

It was Friday. He told me he intended to get a lipid panel done on Monday. I told him this was not conclusive and gave him the phone number for his doctor to order the HeartStopper test kit as a follow-up. With our history, there was no time to waste. He needed to know his small-particle status. We rang off and I sat staring out the window. What had I done? A young couple expecting their first child suddenly had their world turned on its head.

I told Beverly how stupid I felt for not approaching the topic more slowly, for not softening the blow.

She said, "Honey, you probably just saved his life."

I could hope.

CHAPTER 9

Memories

Right after my father died, one of his partners told me that my father had complained of pain in his left arm and a little dizziness hours before he had come home. The year was 1970. The advertisement of a heart attack's warning signs was not as widespread as it is today. If my father or one of the other cops hadn't been in the middle of a riot, maybe somebody would have put two and two together and dragged him to a hospital. He might have lived. Instead, he came home and collapsed on the kitchen floor, dead almost instantly.

I remember how angry I was at him for leaving my mother a widow and me and my younger brother to finish growing up without him.

He had recently resumed smoking. I blamed him for that.

He had ignored signs of a heart attack. I blamed him for that.

He'd had gallbladder surgery only two months earlier and was not in peak physical condition to return to work. I blamed him for that.

For years and years I was angry at a dead man for not taking better care of himself and for depriving us of the twenty or thirty years he should have had left to live.

Now I realize he never had a chance. At least he had made it to fifty. I barely survived my gene-induced heart attack at forty-five. Medical science has only recently recognized the existence of heart-killer genes. Testing for our condition began only a few years ago.

It's ironic that I could forgive my father for what in my youth I thought were his health transgressions only after I had been struck down by the genes he carried. I don't blame him for giving them to me.

CHAPTER 10

Revenge

It was time for revenge. The Lasix in my IV had been a low blow. It had ruined a night's sleep, and sleep is an all too precious commodity in the hospital where one is being stabbed and squeezed and shocked and zapped randomly at all hours of the day and night.

The shift had changed before dinner. The same crew as the previous night was on board in the ICU. One of the nurses came in and checked my vital signs.

"You know, dinner wasn't that great tonight," I said.

"Oh, really?"

"Why don't you look surprised?"

The nurse gave me a wry grin.

"The cafeteria's open twenty-four hours, isn't it?" I said it casually. "I just might have to go down there."

"Dream on," she said with a chuckle.

"No, I really would like some fat-free frozen yogurt. Something cool. I'm a little hot."

"Your temp is fine."

"Yeah, well, I feel hot."

I had planted a seed. Now it was time to make it grow.

When the nurse had been gone a few minutes, I got out of bed and disconnected my cardiac monitor from the jack in the wall. Wheeling my portable IV stand, I shuffled out of my room and up the hall away from the nurses' station. It was still during visiting hours; civilians were wandering the halls. Camouflage. Using a knot of family members moving toward the elevators, I headed for the lounge, found a recent Sunday *New York Times,* and propped it in front of me. I began reading book reviews.

In about one minute, I heard voices raised around the corner.

I heard my name a couple of times. Most of it I couldn't make out, but at one point I heard the word *cafeteria*. I hunkered down in my chair and kept the *Times* in front of me.

After ten minutes, I left the lounge and peeked around the corner toward my room. The hall was clear. I shuffled the fifty feet to my room as quickly as I could. I reconnected my cardiac monitor in the wall. As I climbed into bed, my heart was racing from the exertion of moving quickly. As I heard the drumming of my pulse in my ears, I had a sudden fear that this prank would be my undoing. What a price to pay for a practical joke! I arranged my covers, flicked off the lights, and stretched quietly in my bed, willing my heart to slow its frenzied beating.

I absently rubbed my sternum. It never stopped itching. It was all I could do to keep from ripping my nails into my skin to find relief. My chest had been the battleground of life and death, and like any battleground after the combatants had left the field, it carried the scars of that struggle. My first- and second-degree burns were a splotchy red reminder of the voltages that had coursed through me. The underlying bones of the sternum had not been broken during CPR compressions, but they had been flexed to their limits, leaving behind a dull, constant ache to go with the itching. It would be six months before these bones would heal. On top of that, the ER staff had shaved me from throat to groin, and the emerging stubble only added to the itching. Each day, nurses tore off the half dozen two-inch, plastic adhesive patches that connected electrodes from my chest to my heart monitor and replaced them, never in quite the same locations. This daily trauma pulled out my reemerging chest hairs and aggravated my burned skin again and again. To this day, the hair on my chest has not grown back to anything near its former coverage.

I lay in the dark for almost fifteen minutes before the charge nurse sauntered in. As she flicked on the lights, she said, "Where have *you* been?"

I feigned sleepiness and yawned. "Me? I've been right here."

Her brown eyes flashed. "Here? We've been looking all over for you."

"You must have checked the wrong room. I've been right here."

I was so deadpan, she didn't know what to say. In such a large place, it was just remotely possible that what I said was true. She exited, but returned within a minute with the nurse who had checked my vitals. "He says he's been right here."

The new arrival was one of the feistier nurses. She stared right at me. "How was the frozen yogurt?"

I put on a feigned hurt expression. "Yogurt? Now, how could I get yogurt? Nurse, please check the property inventory. You'll see I don't have a wallet with me and I don't have money. How could I possibly buy frozen yogurt?" What my words said was belied by my tone. I wanted her to know I was playing with her.

"How'd you get down there? We looked all over the cafeteria."

"Nurse, you know I'm too weak to go anywhere. And I wouldn't think of going to the cafeteria without the wheelchair guy. That would be against the rules." My eyes were wide.

"Do you realize what—"

I cut her off by clutching my chest. "Nurse, you're stressing me. Do you want to be the cause of my second heart attack?"

Her eyes automatically went to the monitor above my head. "You're fine."

"Yes, but the stress of this browbeating could put me over." I held the back of my right hand against my forehead in my best impression of a fainting Scarlett O'Hara and said, "Oh, I'm feeling weak." I fluttered my lashes at them.

The charge nurse looked at the other woman. "Is he always like this?"

The other said, "No, he's usually worse."

I quickly interjected, "Yeah, those side effects. Lasix makes me a little cranky. That's why I shouldn't get it too often." I looked pointedly at the feisty one.

She squinted and then started to laugh.

Meaningfully I said, "I'll be good if you'll be good."

"Deal."

I was glad for the truce. This was getting nuts.

THE BLACK RUBBER SUBMARINE

After all the probing, prodding, sticking, zapping, and other handling I had endured, I thought I had become jaded. How wrong I was.

Toward the end of my first week in the hospital, I was informed that my doctors wanted to do a *trans-esophageal echocardiogram*. Some mouthful, right? I had no idea what a mouthful really was until they prepped me for this one. The echocardiograms I had received up to this point were simple: they spent maybe twenty minutes moving a high-frequency sound probe over my chest and recorded the echo images of my heart. Very much like the sonogram that shows a woman her fetus so that doctors can assess the baby's development, this was a sonogram that showed my beating heart so that specialists could interpret how much it had been damaged.

The "esophageal" part was the new twist. For this sonogram, they had to get the sound probe down my throat.

The external sonograms I'd had were hampered by having to project sound waves through skin and fat and ribs and lungs; a lot of body tissue was blocking accurate images. Since the esophagus passes right by the heart, putting a probe down my throat would enable the doctors to get a really clear picture of my heart, with almost nothing to block the sound waves.

Now, when they told me about a "probe," my mind formulated a picture of some thin, fiber-optic miracle that would snake down my throat. I had no preparation for what really was to happen.

A team of two nurses and one doctor wheeled an electronics-laden cart into my room. It was the now-familiar echo machine that was equipped with TV screens to watch the images produced by the sound probe, along with recording equipment to make a videotape for later detailed analysis.

If one just stays quiet on one's bed, I have learned that hospital staff will come in, do their business, and leave with little or no personal interaction with the patient. They're busy and they don't have loads of time. For this reason, I usually do something to get their attention, to say essentially, "Hey, I'm real, I'm alive,

I'm not just a hunk of meat." This group was new to me and particularly efficient, so I was determined to have fun.

As they uncarted wires and tubes and began spinning up their equipment, it looked a little scary. These people *do* things to you.

I said in my best British accent, "Please don't torture me again. Copernicus was *wrong!* The earth does *not* revolve around the sun. The earth is the center of the universe! I recant! Dear God, I recant!"

The nurses were smiling and Beverly, sitting at the other end of the room, started to laugh. But the doctor was a stoic, going about his business with only a weird glance in my direction. Several of the floor nurses gathered near the door to see how the newcomers would handle me, their most fragile yet most difficult patient.

"All right, I *admit* that the earth is flat! I was wrong! I recant! I now truly believe that the Holy Mother Church is the font of all wisdom. Do with me what you will. Bury me in leeches or break me on the rack, but please, I beg of you, allow my family to go free!"

The doctor finally cracked a smile. He said, "Are you *sure* it's flat?"

I nodded vigorously and said in awed tones, "Oh, Holy One, guide me."

I finally got to see his teeth.

One of my floor nurses said to the doctor, "Show him the probe. That'll shut him up."

They did. It shut me up.

They opened a long black box that, I swear, was padded inside with gray velvet. Sitting in this plush setting was a thick black thing about eight inches long. It looked like a black rubber submarine. The doctor set the display box on the cart and grasped a control wire that snaked out of one end of this contraption. He moved the controller and the black rubber submarine started to contort. One end of it rose and twisted around.

My eyes went wide and my mouth went shut. It was like some diabolical puppet. For a chilling moment I thought of the movie *Alien* when the baby alien bursts through the chest of its host and looks around. It looked just like that, sitting in its nice little black and gray coffin.

In a whisper I said, "Now we're *really* going to have some fun."

One of the nurses gave me a shot of anesthetic through my IV. The doctor began explaining the procedure, but I don't remember any of it. All I could do was stare at the black rubber submarine and wonder how in the world they were going to get that thing down my throat. The answer was, of course, drugs. They were going to dope me up to the point where I wouldn't care what they stuck in me. At least that was the theory. What they didn't know was that I metabolized anesthetics rapidly. It was difficult to knock me out.

Everything went fast. I was feeling dopey and hoping they'd all go away when, suddenly, the submarine was out of its box and poised above my face. Jesus, up close it looked like a cop's night-stick. I started to squirm, despite the drugs.

"Whoa, whoa, daddy-o, how the hell does this work?"

The doctor tried to reassure me. "As the drugs kick in, your throat muscles will relax. Your gag reflex will be suppressed. We need you conscious to follow directions for the first part of the procedure, but then you'll drift off. This particular drug will make you forget the whole thing afterwards."

This wasn't reassuring me. "The procedure's that bad that I need to forget it?"

"Well, maybe not that bad."

"Then why do I need to forget it?"

"It goes fast. Don't worry."

It had only been a few days since they had taken the horrible breathing tube out of my trachea. My memories of struggling for every breath for two days were vivid in my mind. Having some-thing even bigger go down my throat was frightening. I took a moment to compose myself and then said, "All right, let's do this."

The doctor put the end of the submarine into my mouth and pushed it to the back of my throat. I thought I should be gagging, but I wasn't. When it felt as if I had swallowed a Buick, the doctor said, "Swallow now."

If I had been able to speak, I would have said, "You gotta be kidding." But instead, I made my throat swallow. It went down and down and I started to panic. This big, hard mass was in the middle of my chest and I thought I wouldn't be able to breathe. I started squirming involuntarily.

"It's okay. We're where we need to be. We're recording. Just a few minutes. Just take it easy." The doctor's voice droned on and on, trying to soothe me.

I tried to let the drug take me away. I tried not to concentrate on the immediacy of the hands in my face and the swooshing, chugging sound of the sonogram. I couldn't see the TV screens, but I could hear the Dopplered sound image. It was a horror show.

This was like a nightmare I once had where I woke up during an operation and the surgeons ignored me. I'm sure this echo team thought I was pretty far gone, but my body fought the drugs and I was fairly lucid. I gripped the sides of the bed and endured as the swooshing sound went on and on.

I opened my eyes and looked around. I saw hands and faces. The faces were watching the TV screen, not me. My face was puffy and bruised, so I don't blame them. But finally one of the nurses looked into my eyes. "You're awake, aren't you?"

I opened my eyes wide in assent. They gave me another shot of something and I drifted off. It was such a relief. I didn't want to be conscious when they pulled that thing out of me.

When I woke up later that afternoon, contrary to what the doctor had told me, I remembered far too much.

My brother, Greg, was sitting next to my bed. When he saw me stir, he began talking as if we had been in the middle of a conversation. "You know, I never could get behind calling you Miracle Man. But now I have a name for you I'm real comfortable with."

"Yeah? What's that?" I croaked.

"Deep Throat."

I threw a pillow at him.

CHAPTER 11

First Night

On the fourteenth day after my hospital incarceration, I was discharged. Amid the well-wishings of the nursing staff I had come to know so well, the ubiquitous wheelchair arrived for me, and my attendant scooped me up. I jokingly gave my royal-family wave to the assembled masses, was wheeled to the exit, and was discharged. The drive home with Beverly and my mother and brother felt like an amusement ride, so unused to car travel had I become. My walk up my driveway to my home was the first time I had been outdoors in two weeks. My skin was pale and I shuffled. I felt as if I had not been home for a hundred years. Now like some traveler returned from wandering the world, needing the solace of the home fires, I hurried to reach the front door.

The sun glowed through the million new leaves that spring had festooned over the withered sticks of winter. The scent of freshly mowed lawns curled through the air. The cacophony of a thousand birds fighting over nesting materials rang through the neighborhood. It was high spring. I hoped my own rebirth would be as successful as that of all around me.

It was strange to enter my house again. The last time I had passed through the front door I had been on a stretcher. It felt like a small victory to make my entrance on my own two feet. Inside there was the evidence of my three family members' habitation—jackets on the backs of chairs, unknown satchels, coffee cups on the dining table—all the hundred tiny testimonials to a normalcy of which I had not been a part.

My dog, Emily, a huge Black Lab–Akita, was a forest of attention. Her normal greeting—lunges into my thighs—was now frenzied, as she had not seen her master for two weeks. Her nudges now felt like hits from the Green Bay Packers line. The booming rumbles that issued from her massive chest would seem, to the outside observer, the precursor to mayhem. But she is a gentle brute and I sat on the floor to let her get it out of her system. It seemed better than getting knocked down.

I was home, yet I felt strange. I suddenly saw the house as nothing but sticks and mortar. I, who had been out among the stars, no longer felt an attachment to place. The people, my family inside the house were important, but the structure I had once taken such pride in no longer mattered to me.

It was strange, too, to be away from the protective womb of the hospital. I missed the familiar weight of the cardiac telemetry monitor in my pocket. For two weeks my every heartbeat, every change in temperature or respiration, every event in my life, had been observed and recorded. At the slightest sign of trouble I had known that a team of skilled medical professionals would be at my side and would make it right. I had become so used to that security I had stopped thinking about it. Now, suddenly, my umbilical was cut. I was on my own. If I felt a twinge in my chest, I couldn't hit the call button to consult with a nurse. Now it was up to me to recognize the difference between muscular pains, indigestion, and true heart difficulty.

Though my family was available for moral support, they could not give me medical opinions. They couldn't look at my electrocardiogram and tell me the status of my heart. Suddenly, in the midst of familiarity, in the place I once associated with security, I felt afraid. I had lost my medical security blanket.

Normally laconic, I had learned in the hospital to discuss my physical symptoms and speculations in great detail with my doctors and nurses. To diagnose me they had needed full information on what was going on inside me, not just from the machines, but through the filter of my perceptions. I tried this with my family. I told them of my concerns. We worked out several strategies on what to do if I felt certain pains or dizziness or weakness. We discussed when it would be necessary to call an ambulance.

It was like practicing for a fire drill. It made me feel less apprehensive. Even if I passed out, people now knew what to do.

Internally, I was undergoing constant change. The massive damage to my heart, apart from changing how my heart beat and functioned, had also changed the electronic "wiring" of my heart. My electrocardiogram (EKG) looked very different from a normal person's. Not only was it different from normal, it became different from itself over time. It was scary to watch my EKG change from week to week as my heart readjusted to its new, limited capabilities. To keep beating, it had to reroute nerve impulses. Its timing changed.

Scar tissue was forming and would continue to form for months. Blood pressure would try to expand the damaged walls of my heart and push them out like a balloon. If this happened, I would become weaker as my heart enlarged. If my heart got too big, it would become inefficient and I would likely develop congestive heart failure. It would take six months for my heart to stabilize. In that time I would be constantly alert to every twitch and pain I felt in my chest.

Also, there was a 30 percent chance that the area in the coronary artery that had blocked might close down again. Angioplasty did not always succeed in keeping a constricted artery open. It might be necessary to install a stent, a tiny tube, at the site of the close-down to keep the artery open. Other arteries might also become clogged. At this time in my treatment, nobody was looking for a heart-killer gene. The immediate goal was to deal with the effects of the heart attack and to keep me alive. Nobody yet knew of the propensity my body had for clogging its arteries.

So, having overcome incredible odds, I did not feel triumphant. I knew I was only beginning the second act of a three-act play. The curtain could come down any moment and end my performance.

Through the rest of that first day, we all relaxed. Being outside the hospital was a signal that things were better, that I was more stable. We joked and laughed and stayed up too late. I forgot my fears for a while and finally was too tired to worry. I had made it through First Day, now I had to face my First Night.

That first night I discovered how dependent I had become on the adjustable hospital bed. In my own bed I could only lie flat, which soon became uncomfortable. As soon as I got horizontal, either on my back or my side, I began to have PVCs (premature ventricular contractions). These out-of-rhythm contractions scared the bejesus out of me. Even though my cardiologist had told me they were not dangerous unless they ran on and on, I didn't want to feel even one. The heart attack was still too fresh in my mind for me to allow any kind of offbeat thumping in my chest.

After experimenting with all sorts of supports, I settled on using two sofa cushions and a pillow behind me to prop me up to about a forty-five-degree angle. It would be a terrible way to sleep.

As I kept rearranging my cushions and fidgeting, Beverly leaned over from her side of the bed and began rubbing my neck. She knows this relaxes me. She snuggled closer and as she reached under my neck with one arm, leaned down, and kissed me.

I had showered and shaved a few hours earlier in celebration of being released from all the restrictions of the hospital, where I had felt like a disheveled, greasy, hairy brute. For the first time in two weeks I felt that I was actually kissable. I joined in whole-heartedly with my woman's ministrations.

Beverly and I had been under constant scrutiny in the hospital. We both realized that we were now alone in my bed. Despite having been together in the hospital, we had been little more than roommates. Suddenly we realized how much we had missed being alone together. What had been a loving show of affection began to heat up.

From the drugs and the sleep deprivation of the hospital and the weakness, I was half-dizzy as my pulse increased, so I don't remember how she did it, but somehow, she shucked us out of our pajamas in record time. Released from the horrible restriction of my cloth prison, I reveled in our nakedness. Her body felt like a furnace as she pressed demandingly into me.

The thing I feared and the thing I wanted became sudden reality. We were making love. Part of my mind was recoiling with the fear of what this activity would do to me. As my heart raced, I could hear every beat, could imagine clots forming, tissue tearing, envision all manner of train-wreck images within my chest.

The other part of my mind was brimming with the life force that union with Beverly always generates. I had faced down death, and if I could not celebrate life with the one being I had returned from the void to be with, then what was the point of remaining on earth? It seemed like eternities that we had been separate.

We attacked each other as if we had each been alone for years. All the fear and anxiety of the past two weeks fueled this backlash of emotion. We did not want to be afraid. We did not want to live with me as a fragile egg carton. We wanted our old life together. We coalesced into a thrumming union of spirit and flesh. Triumphant energies coursed through us. For a while, time ceased to have meaning.

Afterward, my weakness was in direct proportion to the fierceness of my exertions. I was exhausted. It took only minutes to fall asleep. The last thing I remember was holding Beverly's hand as I repositioned myself on my cushion mountain.

Only months later did I learn what the rest of the night had been like for Beverly. She was mortified that she had attacked me on my first night home. Every few minutes she checked to make sure I was breathing. Though she had wanted me desperately, she felt that the price she would pay for her wantonness was my death. She barely slept the rest of that night as she flayed herself with recriminations over her weakness and kept a constant vigil on my rising and falling chest.

I awoke happy as a clam to Beverly's haggard visage. I thought it so sweet how she napped through most of the following day. I saw it as her being drained from our lovemaking. Little did I realize the true cause of her exhaustion. Such are the blind spots of the male ego.

When she finally told me her side of the story, months later, we both laughed hysterically. She had no idea how therapeutic our first night together had been for me. Far from being a threat to my health, it had reinvigorated my will to live.

Heart attack and sex, weirdly enough, are intertwined. To almost die makes one very aware of the limited life that may remain. My desire for both deeper emotional and physical intimacy with my soon-to-be-wife was very much the result of my near-death experience.

At the same time it becomes more important, sexual intimacy also becomes somewhat frightening. Who hasn't heard the apocryphal stories about men dying in the middle of making love, leaving their wives or lovers with the horror of suddenly occupying a bed with a corpse? The most terrible story I remember reading was about a heavy man who had a heart attack while making love with his wife, leaving her pinned under him for hours until neighbors heard her shouts and called the police. The poor woman was emotionally scarred for life after almost suffocating under her dead husband.

Morbid? Yes. But it's something men think about.

The first time making love after a heart attack is like Caesar crossing the Rubicon. It is not done without trepidation, soul-searching, and fear.

It continues to be a burr in the mind. One always thinks, "Is this the last time?"

I think that this is a much larger issue for men than for women. From puberty onward, men define themselves in terms of their sexuality. First comes the teen discovery of this thing between our legs that becomes a driving force in our lives. Then come the twenties when most men see themselves as sexual conquistadors, searching not so much for quality as quantity. In our thirties, many men shift into a quest for quality: that one woman who will be a soul mate. As middle age approaches, fears of impotence and old age arise and a man either becomes more deeply involved with his mate or he suddenly seeks more nubile flesh to make him feel young again. For some men, it sometimes becomes, once again, a numbers game.

A heart attack merely intensifies whatever course a man is on, throwing in this new, risky variable. However, this fear is more about perception than fact.

I now know that the chances of dying during lovemaking are slim. An article in a recent medical publication put the odds of dying during sex at about one in 2 million. How they compute such things is beyond me, but it was reassuring to read. The reality is that if one exercises regularly and has built up cardiac strength and efficiency, there is no more reason to fear love-making than a session at the health club. Actually, my health club seems far more dangerous: one can be trampled by weight lifters in the occasional stampede to get at the newest machine.

CHAPTER 12

Cold Reality

Through most of my life, up until my heart attack, I was usually in good spirits. At work, people have always asked me why I'm so happy as I whistle down the halls. I have seldom felt down.

But now I am nagged by my mortality, by the clear realization that some portion of my life has been lopped off. Five years, ten? I don't know the number. When I moved to Reno, Nevada, two months after my heart attack, in my first interview with my new cardiologist, Dr. Frank Carrea, he did what I am sure he was trained to do: he didn't overly arouse my expectations. He had a sober discussion with me about my survival chances.

Dr. Carrea started out by telling me about the damage my heart had sustained. It was substantial. The front wall of the left ventricle was "dead." This caused some distortion to the functioning of the mitral valve and the tricuspid valve. Damage to the left ventricle also caused a moderate amount of regurgitation within my heart. Simply put, when my heart pumped, instead of all the blood flowing out the left ventricle to the body, some of it pushed back into the heart, causing back pressure. The invisible result is that the regurgitating blood has the potential to form tiny micro-clots within the heart at the apex of the left ventricle.

Grim? Yes. I had never had such a sobering conversation. Carrea then put my survival in these terms: "Your five-year survival potential is eighty-five to ninety-five percent. That's very good." Of course, I saw it from a very different perspective. What I heard was that I had a 5 to 15 percent chance of dying within five years.

Long term, he put it like this: "Most men your age can expect to live into their seventies. You shouldn't expect that. It's possible, but you would have to be very lucky."

Seeing my alarm, he continued, "There's no way to quantify this. I wouldn't go out and quit my job and spend all my money. You're not facing something imminent. But I can't put a number on this for you. Will you live thirty more years? Probably not. Will you live twenty more years? There's a good chance of that. It depends on how you eat, how much you exercise, your general lifestyle."

Nobody knows when death will pounce. I certainly don't, but I strongly suspect that I won't live as long as I might have. Somewhere between tomorrow and maybe twenty years from now, my heart will weaken and I will face a downward spiral. My cardiologist put it this way: "I want to know if you have difficulty breathing when you lie down. It could mean the beginnings of congestive heart failure. If your heart becomes weaker, it can't pump all the fluids through your body. Your lungs will begin to fill with fluid. Many patients go this route. Some sooner, some later. If it happens, we have to start thinking about a heart transplant if there's time."

This is mind-boggling. The thought of having to wait for someone else to die to get his heart; to be on a waiting list hoping for someone with the right tissue match to fall off a building or crash in a car, to experience something bad enough to kill him, but not bad enough to damage his heart; then to have to undergo probably the most radical surgery known to medicine, with no guarantee that the new heart will take, will not be rejected for the foreign tissue that it is? This is my future? Part of me thinks it would be better to die when that day comes. Just slip off to that quiet place I have experienced before, rather than undergo the horror of a heart transplant. I'm sure that if I am finally faced with this prospect, I will be less willing to slip away. I'll probably want to continue the fight and I'll let them cut me open and I'll live with the huge rehab prospect afterward.

Or what if I start to throw clots from the regurgitation in my heart? What if one goes to my brain and I have a stroke, becoming a vegetable? This is my worst nightmare: to be trapped in my body the same way as when I first awoke after my heart attack, paralyzed now from something irreversible rather than from the drug they had given me to stop my seizures.

I wonder that I am not depressed all the time. Somehow I can usually keep myself from dwelling on these thoughts, from dreading the future. But every so often, I become maudlin and my mood turns sour. I become irritable. I am sure I am not a pleasure to be around. At those times, I retreat into a private world and I read a book or I write. I'm sure for some heart patients, therapy would be helpful. I have not yet been able to cross that bridge. I cope with my occasional bouts of depression as I have all my life, locked in an internal dialogue until a path through the brambles emerges. Exercise helps.

My goal is to stay as healthy as I can, to live well in the time I have left. Dr. Carrea told me after the first year under his care that he was surprised I had not been back in the hospital. He said that many patients in my condition were back in the hospital every so often with breathing problems and arrhythmias. He attributes my continued good health to the fact that I exercise religiously.

Recently he told me that I was probably more physically fit than most men my age. This is encouraging and keeps me going to the gym at least four days a week.

It also makes me realize how easy it is to feel sorry for oneself and to slip into a longer-term depression. This is a self-fulfilling trap. Feel bad, stop exercising, eat some chocolate to feel better. A few months of that and the whole body weakens to the point that trouble becomes inevitable. It's a one-way trip to the ER.

How to stay away from that route? In the following chapters, I delve more closely into the causes of this disease and what can be done to prevent its destructive effects. For those who may already have survived a heart attack, we are in the same boat. I hope the approach I have taken may be helpful to you. If I can come back from the dead after suffering severe damage to my heart, then there is hope for others, too.

CHAPTER 13

The Wrong Stuff

Around the sixth day after my heart attack, after I had weaned myself off oxygen, my cardiologist suggested I try getting out of bed and sitting in a chair for half an hour or so. He told me I had lost 85 percent of my body strength. He was concerned that staying in bed would weaken my heart further. I agreed, since I felt incredibly weak compared to my physical condition before the MI.

The first time I got into a chair, it was an ordeal. I couldn't move well and had to be helped. It was embarrassing. I felt like an old man. At forty-six, I could go no farther than the bedside chair because I was wired up to heart-monitoring equipment that looked remarkably like the medical displays on the original *Star Trek*.

After a couple days, I was able to get out of bed by myself and spent hours reading or watching television while sitting up. The difference of body position put more stress on my heart, but also made it marginally stronger.

After ten days in ICU, I was considered well enough to move to a telemetry ward. The ever-present electrodes on my chest were hooked to leads from a portable heart monitor about the size of a pack of cigarettes. This fit into the pocket of my hospital gown and transmitted my heart status to the nurses' station, where someone monitored the telemetry screens twenty-four hours a day. If something bad started to happen to my heart, the nurses would immediately know.

The advantage was that I was no longer tethered to my bed by wires. I could get up and move around. We all take for granted the simple task of going to the bathroom, but if one has spent over a week in bed, forbidden to use the bathroom or shower, that first trip is a small piece of heaven.

The nurses encouraged me to try short walks. "Walk" was a misnomer. I shuffled. I learned how quickly a seemingly healthy body could go downhill. I had almost no strength and even a short walk left me winded. I had lost fifteen pounds.

My second day in the telemetry unit dawned to a surprise. Around 9 A.M. a nurse appeared at my door with a wheelchair. "We're going to rehab. Today you exercise."

I thought it bizarre that I would be taken by wheelchair to exercise. "Why not walk there if I need exercise?"

"We don't want anything to happen to you."

"What can happen to me in the hall that can't happen in the gym?"

"Don't be difficult."

One of my more "difficult" tricks was slowing my heart. I found that by simple meditation, I was able to get my heart rate down to about fifty beats per minute. The average heart rate is around seventy beats per minute. Most damaged hearts beat much faster than that as they speed up to do the same work as before their damage. So when I slowed to fifty beats, I usually got a rise out of the duty nurses, who would scramble into my room to find me quietly watching my heart monitor. "Watch this," I would say, and right before their eyes I'd send my heart rate up to ninety by clenching my feet and leg muscles unseen under the covers.

So, Mr. Difficult or not, I had to learn that to go anywhere in the hospital, I would be transported by wheelchair. No matter that in rehab they would sweat me, push me, prod me to struggle through my paces; in the halls I would be chauffeured like the invalid I didn't want to be.

When they got me to the rehab gym, they spent fifteen minutes telling me what they would do and warning me to tell someone if I felt dizzy or had pains or was disoriented or felt weak. The list went on and on and I began to think that maybe I should just go back to my room. These people clearly thought they might kill me.

Finally, they put me on a treadmill and started it up. I cannot believe what a ridiculous figure I was. Wearing a blue hospital gown, which, even with the strings tied in back, provided scant cover for my rear end, clad in some weird blue socks that had adhesive strips on the bottom for traction, with two black eyes and a face that looked like a nightmare of bruises, here I was shuffling along on a moving rubber belt at a speed normally seen only in K Mart shoppers.

I almost got flung off the treadmill because it started too fast. The nurse/trainer/torturer dialed the controls back, but it was still too fast. She fiddled with it until she got the speed down to .7 mph. To give you an idea of how slow this is, a ninety-year-old with a walker and a hip cast could have whistled by me with ease.

Within five minutes, I was huffing and puffing and begging for mercy. They kept me at it for ten minutes, after which I became grateful for the wheelchair to return me to my room.

Every day they wheeled me up to rehab to prance along on the treadmill, my ass flashing passersby in the hall. By the end of my second week in the hospital I was up to a flaming one mile per hour. As pathetic as this seemed to me, I did feel better.

As weak as I was, my doctor felt I was ready for discharge. Of course, out came the wheelchair for my final journey down the halls. But in those last hours, they exposed me to the plan for the next six weeks: Cardiac Rehab. Three days per week, I was scheduled to return to the rehab gym. They were going to build me up to a semblance of my former self. Though I knew I had to do it, I also knew I had a long way to go. I was not thrilled with the prospect.

After two weeks of being with the ICU patients whose hearts had just turned on them, I was exposed to the general population via Cardiac Rehab. These were the veterans. Some had endured chest pains for years. Others had undergone bypass surgeries. All were older than I.

I was scheduled for morning sessions on Mondays, Wednesdays, and Fridays. Cardiac Rehab 1 was a combination of exercise therapy, counseling, and stress management training. It was a well-balanced approach to overall health.

After several weeks of Cardiac Rehab, I was feeling much

stronger. I could do all the exercises and the nursing staff kept ratcheting my performance level higher. My treadmill speed was now over two miles per hour. I was feeling confident and hopeful that I would not be an invalid.

Then I met a patient I will call Bob. Bob was a big man, about five feet eleven inches and weighing at least three hundred pounds. He looked to be in his late fifties. He always wore denim bib coveralls.

Bob huffed and puffed his way through rehab, clearly not enjoying himself. He grumbled constantly. He didn't want to be there. He was always accompanied by his wife, a thin, birdlike woman whose face showed she was worried about her husband. I'm sure she was the only reason Bob attended rehab. She sat in the visitors' waiting area at the edge of the gym and seldom took her eyes off Bob.

Bob had not had a heart attack, but he had severe arterial blockage that caused chest pain and irregular heartbeats. Bob had to drop at least a hundred pounds or he was headed for serious trouble.

Meeting Bob was a seminal event in my rehabilitation. He was like a bucket of cold water in the face. Seeing him and hearing his story made me very clear on what I must not do. I knew I had to stick with the program or I could become Bob.

The shocking aspect about Bob was his absolute denial of what was happening to him. The reason Bob wore bib overalls was so that the suspender part of the garment could hold a small, portable heart monitor. This device constantly recorded the performance of Bob's heart. Whenever he felt a strange heart rhythm or had a twinge, he would press a button on the monitor, which would save the event for later analysis by Bob's cardiologist. Inside Bob's chest, he had already had a portable defibrillator surgically implanted. This amazing internal device (roughly the size of an old-time pocket watch) monitored Bob's heartbeat; if it sensed arrhythmia, it sent an electrical shock to his heart and got it back on track. For Bob this device was not just a godsend and a miracle, it allowed him to continue to deny his problem.

Once Bob got the portable defibrillator, he didn't have to

worry about his diet. Hell, the machine fixed his heart when it got out of whack. Zap, a little jolt and everything was okay again. Pass the french fries, please.

The problem was that by contriving to avoid a needed behavior change, Bob only weakened his heart more. The defibrillator was an artificial crutch that bought him time, which he squandered.

The really shocking element of the story was supplied by Beverly, who accompanied me to rehab and who also sat in the visitors' waiting area. Chatting with other anxious wives, Bob's wife found out that my fiancée, Beverly, was a registered dietician. She immediately bombarded Beverly with questions about what Bob could and should eat.

In our nutrition classes we had been told that we had to limit our consumption of meat to six ounces of lean meat or fish per day. Six ounces is about one medium-sized chicken breast. The recommended practice was to save up one's fat allowance and have meat at dinner along with other foods in order to feel full and to get through the evening. Six ounces. Once a day. That was it. I took it as gospel.

Bob's wife (I'll call her Anne) asked Beverly, "Is it okay for my husband to have some sausage at breakfast?"

Beverly said, "As long as it's lean sausage, that should be okay." Of course, Beverly was thinking that Anne was asking about the one meal of the day when we were allowed to have meat. For Bob, Beverly was thinking that breakfast would be the meal at which he indulged. Beverly added, "Just make sure it's only six ounces. Just that one time."

Anne looked perplexed. "What do you mean? Just one time?"

Beverly, thinking the woman hadn't understood her, repeated herself. "He can have sausage at breakfast if that's the one meal of the day where he has it. And not too much."

Anne's face brightened as she saw what Beverly was getting at. "Oh, no. He has meat at lunch and dinner; he just wanted to know if he could have it at breakfast, too. He misses it so. Bob sure loves his sausage."

Beverly's mouth hung open in surprise. When she told me of

the exchange after class, I shook my head. "What is Bob thinking? Not having sausage at breakfast is going to cure his heart disease? This is his big sacrifice to save his life?"

Anne had also told Beverly how Bob hated exercise. Anne tried to get him to take walks with her at home, but he refused.

Two weeks later, Bob climbed down off the treadmill in class, wheezing and complaining of dizziness. He was ecstatic when the staff told him he didn't have to exercise any more that day. He trundled out and we never saw him again. A few days later we heard he'd had a heart attack and was in ICU.

Within a short time I finished my rehab course and said good-bye to Mercy Hospital. I don't know what happened to Bob. I'm not too hopeful about his prognosis. It didn't have to happen that way.

Bob wasn't the only one in denial; he was just the worst.

One day in nutrition class, the instructor was telling us about egg-substitute products like Egg Beaters. One of my classmates, a sixtyish man with gray hair, also overweight, said, "Y'know, my wife and I looked at them things at the store. That stuff is expensive."

The nutritionist said, "As a less expensive alternative, you could use regular eggs and separate the yolks. The yolks have the cholesterol. Just use the egg whites."

The man's wife chimed in, "We did that, but them whites don't have much taste. He wouldn't eat 'em."

The nutritionist said, "You could separate maybe five egg whites, then stir in one complete egg for flavor. It would make two servings." It seemed a reasonable compromise. One dose of cholesterol instead of six.

The wife shot back, "I did that, but he still wouldn't eat it. I had to add back three more yolks before it tasted good."

The poor nutritionist was squirming. She clearly wanted to jump all over this couple, but she refrained because when she fought these stout, stubborn farmers, they just stopped coming to class. Seeing his wife had given them the upper hand in the nutrition wars, the husband added, "Them Egg Beaters is too damn expensive."

Several of the other classmates made sounds of agreement.

One of them chimed in, "You always pay for convenience." He had a triumphant look on his face as other heads nodded and grunts of approval rippled through the class. His statement solidified the issue for these farmers and descendants of farmers who had pinched pennies all their lives. None of them wanted to pay for expensive, newfangled, fat-free foods.

In a class of a dozen male patients, most of whom had experienced heart attacks, I felt like the class brownnoser. I was the only one who followed the nutrition recommendations, the only one who didn't fight over every fat gram with the instructor. I didn't do this because I wanted to be the teacher's pet. I did it because I was scared to death. I looked at each morsel of food as a potential fat bomb that would detonate inside my chest.

I sat there mesmerized by the hostility in that classroom. Nobody wanted to change anything. Several of these men had undergone bypass surgery. They saw bypass as the solution. Eat like a hog until your arteries clogged up, get the arteries replaced, and get back to the trough. They refused to hear that in a few years their new coronary arteries would clog right back up and they'd be facing another operation or worse.

They seemed to take pleasure in the group dynamic of sticking together against this foolish young nutritionist. It was like watching a junior high school class take advantage of a substitute teacher. They ganged up on the nutritionist, looking for any chink in her armor. When they found one, they picked at that spot, taking turns refuting the logic of something they did not want to hear. It was mob mentality gone hopelessly awry.

Robert A. Heinlein defined a mob as a dozen stomachs with no brain. Clearly, in this group, the stomachs were the victors.

CHAPTER 14

Oops!

About halfway through my second week in the hospital, I was taken to radiology for a thallium stress test. The purpose of this test is to get a more detailed look at one's heart than is possible with an echocardiogram. I was injected with a radioactive dye that settles in the heart and is picked up by radiophotography sensors. I was then stretched out on a table while a huge sensing device slowly rotated around my upper body, taking cross-sectional images of my heart that would later be assembled by a computer into a three-dimensional image of my heart. The whole process took about a half hour. The most difficult part of it was lying perfectly still for the duration.

Then I was taken to another room where I was hooked up to an EKG and a pulse monitor. A blood pressure cuff was strapped to my arm, and I was put on a treadmill. The technicians explained that once my heart rate was elevated, they would inject more radioactive dye and take another three-dimensional picture of my heart to show how it functioned under stress.

I was told to walk as fast as I could. I slowly built up to my top speed of less than one mile per hour and strained to go faster. I could feel my heart pounding, a small worry; but since I was in the hospital, I figured if anything started to go wrong, someone was immediately available to help me. So I pushed on.

The technicians inclined the treadmill so I was scaling the equivalent of a steep hill. I watched my pulse rate go up to eighty beats per minute, then ninety. Then almost to a hundred. When it hit a hundred, I couldn't go any faster. I was sweating madly and my head hurt. This was the most exercise I'd gotten since my heart attack.

"Can't you go any faster?" the technician asked.

"Not unless you want to kill me," I replied through gritted teeth.

The technician left for a minute and brought in someone else. They conferred over my chart and the monitor that showed my heart rate, blood pressure, and EKG.

One of them turned to me. "You sure you can't go any faster?"

By now my skin was red and I was soaked. By luck I asked the right question. "How fast are you trying to get me?"

"At least one twenty, maybe one thirty."

"A hundred thirty beats per minute?" I was stunned. "That *will* kill me. I'm on a beta-blocker!"

Both technicians looked as if I'd punched them in the face. One shook his head.

I added, "The fastest I can go is about a hundred beats per minute. That's it. Didn't anyone tell you this?"

From the looks on their faces, it was obvious that nobody had.

I was at some risk pushing myself like this. A beta-blocker is a chemical designed to slow one's heartbeat, to make the heart more efficient and less likely to injure itself by racing. My top-end exercise range was eighty to one hundred beats per minute. No matter how much I exercised, the beta-blocker would keep my heart at a slow, efficient rate. I began to slow down as I realized what had happened. Somehow, the crucial piece of information that I was on a beta-blocker had not been communicated with my lab orders.

The point of this story is that people make mistakes. If you have a cold or a broken leg, a mistake won't be fatal. When you have a damaged heart and carry a heart-killer gene, mistakes are much more critical. In my case the radiology technicians hadn't been informed that I was on a beta-blocker and that no amount of physical exercise would stress my heart enough for their test. Once I told the technicians about the beta-blocker, they switched to an alternative means to increase my heart rate, using a chemical called Persantine, which a doctor injected into me.

As I laid on a table waiting for the Persantine to work, I suddenly felt scared. I realized how close I had come to real danger because someone had made a mistake. I was only ten days removed from my heart attack and was being subjected to risks I didn't understand. I raised my head and said to the doctor who was standing next to me, "Doctor, just what is this Persantine?"

I grilled him on how it worked, what results he expected, and anything else I could think of. I found that I could have a life-threatening allergic reaction to Persantine. This was why he had asked me if I was allergic to shellfish just before he injected me. Every way I turned it seemed there was some fatal consequence of a mistake, and I was not being sufficiently briefed on the risks beforehand.

This incident changed my perspective. I learned to ask all medical staff with whom I came in contact what they wanted to do to me, why they wanted to do it, what the risks were, and what they expected as an outcome. I had to be the one to catch the mistakes. I couldn't rely on the system to do it.

We take a huge risk when we offer ourselves into other people's care and then assume they know what to do. The individuals may have all the skills in the world, but they are part of a system that is large and unwieldy. It's better not to assume that everyone coming into contact with you as the patient is knowledgeable about your case.

A year later, another memorable moment occurred while I was getting prepped for gallbladder surgery at Washoe Medical Center in Reno, Nevada. I was reclining on a gurney in the holding area just outside the doors to the surgical theater. Behind me was a long line of other patients on other gurneys. It was like an airport runway clogged with rush-hour flights waiting for take-off. Beverly was with me. We chatted quietly, waiting for something to happen. I was already an hour late for surgery.

Suddenly, a haggard surgeon in greens and a white laboratory coat hurried toward us through the big double doors. He looked ancient, yet he moved with manic energy. Clipboard at the ready, he homed in on me like a Stinger missile.

"You are?" he clipped.

"Bayan."

He consulted his charts. "Oh, yes. You're getting a pacemaker."

A jolt of pure electricity, surpassed only by my experience with the defibrillator, seared through me. My pulse started racing and a thin sweat erupted all over my body. Nobody had told me I needed a pacemaker! Where was my cardiologist?

I shot a glance at Beverly. Her blue eyes looked like a deer's caught in the headlights of an onrushing truck. Our silent communion said, "What rabbit hole have we fallen into?"

After a year of surviving the sometimes Mad Hatter atmosphere of hospitals, I rallied my thoughts. Back to basics. I did what I had learned always to do in these situations: ask questions.

"Doctor, you have orders for me for a pacemaker?" Nothing happened in the hospital without orders.

He flipped through the papers on his clipboard. "Now, what's your name again?" Perplexity pulled at the creases of his face.

"Bayan. Doctor, I'm supposed to have my gallbladder removed."

Now his face really contorted as the papers on his clipboard riffled like leaves in a windstorm.

"Bayan? Bayan? Oh, yes. Okay. Gallbladder."

Without another word of explanation, he scurried behind us to the next gurney, where his now agitated voice said, "Are *you* the pacemaker?" He was a man in a hurry. Not the Mad Hatter; he was more like the White Rabbit, pressed for time, always late.

A half hour later I was stretched out on an operating table. As a gowned and masked nurse prepped me for surgery and started my anesthesia drip, I asked, "This is for my gallbladder removal, right?" The nurse smiled and nodded her head. I closed my eyes and fell under the effects of the anesthesia. My last thought was that I was pretty sure I wouldn't wake up with a pacemaker in my chest. Pretty sure.

CHAPTER 15

New Beginnings

When I regained consciousness after my heart attack, I could not speak because of the respirator tube stuck down my throat. I had a lot of time to think of what I had experienced. I could feel the winds of space so close. I knew that if I did not stay focused on the here and now, I could easily slip back across that thin barrier and leave my life behind.

The first thing I said to Beverly after the doctor took out my breathing tube was, "All your hopes, dreams, and aspirations can be gone in an instant. We're all exactly one heartbeat away from death."

We spend so much of life planning. We defer gratification. We think we will live forever. It just isn't so.

More than once during my two-week hospital stay I almost called the chaplain to marry Beverly and me. But some part of me held back, believing that if I did that, it was because I didn't think I would survive. After much soul-searching, I resolved to wait. I now knew clearly that I would not live forever, but I didn't want to do something desperate as if admitting I only had a few days to live.

I waited until I had moved to Reno, Nevada, Beverly's home, to make marriage plans. After settling in, we made rapid arrangements for our wedding.

Now, researchers who study these things say that the big stressors in life are the death of a loved one (I had almost experienced that stress firsthand); moving one's home (yeah, that was in July); getting a new job (July again); and getting married. They say that experiencing any one of these things in a given year is a major life stress and takes a toll. Many people die after such stresses. Since 1996 was already far beyond the normal bounds of any kind of stress measurement, I wanted to cram it all into one year so 1997 would seem like a vacation. So, we set November 9, 1996, as our wedding date. It would be exactly six months after my heart attack. It was a milestone.

I've seen people spend two years planning their weddings. We spread the planning over three months and adopted the Nike approach. We just did it.

On the scheduled date, there we stood, high in the Sierra Nevada on a rocky precipice overlooking Lake Tahoe. Two weeks earlier, a foot of snow had fallen, but on this day, the air was warm, the sky clear, and not a breath of wind stirred the cobalt blue surface of the lake. It was as if having been dealt all the bad luck at once in May, I was now charmed. It felt like a late-summer day. Despite the fact I was a little dizzy at that altitude, it was an exhilarating experience to have an outdoor ceremony in such a stunningly beautiful location. Under that vault of sky-blue pink, Beverly and I said our vows in the company of our closest friends and relatives.

I had survived six months. I was stronger. I believed it was now possible to go on and beat the odds for at least another decade or two. I was now joined with my best friend in the ongoing adventure of life. But I was also the center of a great experiment of nutrition, medication, and exercise. I had a newly discovered genetic disorder and was in uncharted territory. Nobody knew exactly how to treat my disease. I had to take an active role in analyzing the information my doctor gave me, had to weigh various risks and ultimately make the decisions about which courses of treatment made the most sense for me.

CHAPTER 16

One Size Fits All

As surprising as it sounds, many health professionals know nothing about the HeartStopper Effect, because they are still operating inside a strong paradigm that is counterproductive for carriers of heart-killer genes.

A gross example of this can be seen in cardiac rehabilitation programs. Just about every major hospital in the country has cardiac rehab. It is usually broken into three phases. Cardiac Rehab 1 is the basic course. For the freshly damaged, this is the first step back to recovery. This course teaches nutrition and stress management, and one exercises in a gym, usually three times per week. The course usually runs about six weeks.

Phase 2 is another six weeks, in which exercise is stepped up to bring one as close to full function as possible. Patients get more advanced training in diet and stress reduction.

Phase 3, usually optional, is designed to help patients really integrate what they've learned into day-by-day life.

When I first entered phase one, I didn't know what to expect. It was a little daunting to enter a huge gym with a dozen other men I had never met before. Each of us was given a portable cardiac telemetry device, and we were taught how to connect its three electrodes on our chests. In the center of the gym was a bank of computers staffed by two nurses whose job it was to watch our cardiac performance. It was like the cardiac telemetry unit, but here they would stress us. The rhythms on those screens were going to be very different from the ones up in the telemetry unit where everyone was bedridden.

After warm-up exercises, we were each assigned to a treadmill and started off. There were men in their seventies. I had just turned forty-six. But we all did the same things. I expected some kind of individual plan and was surprised at the cattle-call atmosphere.

I learned that the treatment for all patients after a heart attack is basically the same. Therapists put you on a treadmill and start you walking. At first you may only be able to shuffle, so they get you to shuffle. They keep pushing you to higher and higher plateaus of physical effort. First you shuffle, then you walk. Then you walk faster. Then you walk uphill on an incline. It's all designed to incrementally build up your heart muscle again. The goal is simple: to strengthen damaged hearts.

It doesn't matter if one patient has damage to his left ventricle or that another is recovering from quadruple bypass surgery. The treatment is the same: exercise is good for any heart, no matter what its condition. So the one-size-fits-all approach offers no particular danger to any patient. The medical establishment has used this technique on millions of patients. It works. So it is replicated over and over.

Stress reduction? Who won't benefit from cutting down stress in their lives? Again, a no-brainer. One size fits all. So, we worked with an instructor on meditation techniques to relax our minds and on yoga to relax our bodies.

The same has been true with nutrition. Over decades, cardiac medical practitioners have learned that lowering fat and cholesterol intake limits arterial plaque and reduces the risk of heart attacks. When researchers look at the results for a million people, low-fat, low-cholesterol diets generally show benefits.

Here's the problem. Hidden within that million-person sample are thousands of people who have the HeartStopper Effect. For them, exercise and stress reduction are just as beneficial as for all the other cardiac patients. But the one-size-fits-all paradigm is not good in the area of nutrition. For carriers of a killer gene, a diet loaded with carbohydrates triggers a rise in triglycerides and production of deadly small-particle LDL.

I was caught up in this paradigm for three months before I moved to Reno, Nevada, and had my first appointment with Dr. Carrea. During that three-month period, my triglycerides kept rising. I was headed for more trouble *because* I was being treated in the way that had helped so many other heart attack patients. The concepts that had become common practice were doing me no good. And remember, I was being treated by experienced cardiologists in Des Moines.

You will run into resistance when you start talking about LDL small-particle syndrome, or LDL subclass B, or whatever term you want to use to describe this disease. Many doctors don't know anything about it. From the training they received twenty or even five years ago, they believe that a low-fat diet, substituting carbohydrates for fat, is the proper treatment for all heart patients. They need to be persuaded to look at new information. This is your job.

I'm not saying to *not* listen to your doctor. I'm saying listen, but listen well. Make sure you understand what the doctor tells you. If you don't understand, ask questions. Keep asking questions until you do understand. Nobody is better able to defend your interests and your life than you.

If the idea of questioning your doctor is new to you or makes you uncomfortable, consider this: eighty percent of people with coronary artery disease *do not have elevated cholesterol levels!* If 80 percent of the people whose arteries are getting clogged with cholesterol don't have elevated cholesterol levels, doesn't it seem that the standard method of cholesterol testing is missing the mark? In light of this, does looking at a total cholesterol count and saying that a patient is healthy because his count is under 200 make sense? Yet it continues in the face of irrefutable evidence that this standard of diagnosis is woefully inadequate.

I mentioned earlier that roughly 50 percent of all heart attack victims have no knowledge they have heart disease. They just keel over suddenly, not knowing what hit them. How could anyone possibly think that current screening and diagnosis procedures for heart disease are either accurate or successful if 750,000 people each year are unexpectedly waylaid? Something else must be going on inside people's blood systems. Other factors must be at work. To get at these inner disease workings, not only full lipid panels are needed, but also the LDL subclass screenings that get at the subfractions of LDL where HeartStopper genes do their nasty work.

I am in no way suggesting that you should abandon the medical community and go off on your own. My point has been that doctors may not immediately see the genetic component of hyperlipidemia. They may believe you have high cholesterol because of what you eat. You may be overweight and sedentary. It's easy to diagnose run-of-the-mill high cholesterol and to prescribe one-size-fits-all treatments. And if you are among the group whose lipid panel looks better than normal, persuading your doctor to have your LDL subclass analyzed could be difficult. A good lipid panel does not mean the HeartStopper Effect is not present; if you have first-degree relatives who have had heart attacks, the chances you could have a HeartStopper gene are too high to overlook because your lipid panel looks normal.

My message throughout this book is that you must find out if you carry a killer gene because the treatments for the effects of this gene are different from traditional treatments. Small-particle LDL syndrome is a special challenge that requires a different approach for success.

It is possible with lesser ailments to put one's self into a doctor's care and not worry too much about the outcome of treatment. A sprained ankle is a sprained ankle. It's not cancer, it's not emphysema, it's not fatal. But where one's heart is concerned, it is necessary to get involved in the diagnosis and the treatment; to make sure one understands what the doctors are saying.

When was the last time you asked coworkers, friends, and relatives about an issue and heard exactly the same opinion from all of them? It's never happened to me. So, why should we expect the same opinion from different doctors? When you have the potential for a life-threatening illness, you need advice and opinions from more than one medical source. It's called a second opinion, or a third opinion and so on. You must ask and ask until you think you have enough information to make an informed decision.

Patients are confronted with choices every day. Should the woman get a lumpectomy or a mastectomy? Should the man try radiation therapy on his prostate cancer or go for surgery or do nothing at all? Patients can get medical diagnoses and advice, but eventually, they have to make the final decisions. Diagnosis and treatment of a heart-killer gene are no different. Because its existence is not widely understood, it is even more imperative for patients to be alert and vigilant and to be involved in their diagnosis and treatment, sometimes to the point of being rude.

It's disturbing to consider that many doctors are not pressured on this issue because many patients are not even trying to understand and manage their cardiac health. A few years ago, Yankelovich Partners, Inc., one of the largest survey and polling companies in the country, surveyed doctors and patients about blood cholesterol. Pollsters called five hundred patients who were diagnosed as having high cholesterol and two hundred doctors who treat this type of patient. Though most doctors felt they were educating their patients well, three out of four patients did *not* think high cholesterol was a serious health problem. And almost half (42 percent) of them said they weren't concerned about their high cholesterol in the least.

Maybe that's the half that gets the unexpected heart attacks.

CHAPTER 17

Good Health

The secret to good health can be summed up in one word: consistency. The four main components for ongoing cardiac therapy are nutrition, exercise, medication, and stress reduction, but they are worthless without consistency. Forget to take your betablocker and you court disaster. Get lazy and stop exercising, get ready for a trip to the hospital. The cardiac patient lives on a tightrope, but like any good circus performer, if you spend enough time on a tightrope, it becomes home.

In the next few chapters, I outline the regimen I follow. My purpose is to show how it is possible to integrate the various therapies into a normal life. Is my regimen right for you? Possibly not; you have to find your own comfort zone. But I hope this gives you a starting point to make the choices that accommodate your age, weight, and individual needs.

NUTRITION

In counteracting the effects of a killer gene, it's important to understand how to juggle food components. For instance, though this sounds counterintuitive, to reduce cholesterol in the blood, we need fat in our diets. Wait a minute. Aren't we supposed to reduce fat?

Yes and no. Certain fats are beneficial and our goal is to replace damaging fats with helpful fats. But remember earlier when I talked about how I had gone down to a ten-gram fat diet and how my LDL level was not dropping and my triglycerides were rising?

Well, here's where instead of substituting carbohydrates for fat, we substitute fat for fat.

Another chemistry lesson. It's simple to remember and the benefits are great.

In our diets we must deal with three kinds of fat: saturated, polyunsaturated, and monounsaturated.

Saturated fats are abundant in meat, eggs, butter, whole milk, cheese, and many cooking oils. Saturated fats provide the building blocks for bad cholesterol.

Polyunsaturated fats are found in low concentrations in plant products such as grains and beans and in high concentrations in vegetable oils such as corn oil, safflower oil, and margarine.

Monounsaturated fats are found in peanuts and other nuts; avocados; deep-sea fish such as tuna, mackerel, bluefish, salmon, halibut, and swordfish; and in high amounts in canola oil and olive oil.

Suffice it to say that everyone should curtail eating saturated fats, but particularly those of us afflicted with the HeartStopper Effect.

The human body *must* have fat. Fats provide energy and transport fat-soluble vitamins. We cannot function without fat. However, we have choices on the kinds of fats we ingest.

Oils and fats that contain oleic acid are effective in lowering total cholesterol and LDL. These include polyunsaturated fats. Even better are monounsaturated fats.

It appears that fats containing oleic acid are more effective in lowering LDL because they are less susceptible to oxidation. When oil molecules pick up that extra oxygen molecule, they add to the plaque-forming capabilities of LDL. Without oxidation, they lower LDL's deadliness.

My own experience proved this when I actually increased my fat intake (but only with monounsaturates) and watched my LDLs and triglycerides drop dramatically. This does not mean you should run out and hog up on monounsaturated fatty foods. Fat and oil still contain a lot of calories, and if you increase total calories, you will gain weight. The key here is to *replace* saturated fats or excessive carbohydrates with monounsaturated fats, while staying within your total-calorie goal and staying under 30 percent of calories from fat.

The key to managing killer genes is to *continue* eating fats, but to substitute polyunsaturates and particularly monounsaturates (helpful fats) for saturates (harmful fats). This has a double benefit. First, we give our bodies the fats they need for energy. Second, this substitution will lower LDLs and triglycerides. What could be better? And this approach is beneficial to both carriers of the HeartStopper Effect and normal cardiac patients, as well as the general public.

Now, of course, here come the choices: broiled salmon steak versus a Big Mac; a handful of peanuts instead of a handful of potato chips; skim versus whole milk; an orange instead of a candy bar. Yes, we have to change some lifetime habits; the alternative is having no lifetime to change.

Admittedly, this is difficult. The habit component of what people eat is built from early childhood, and unfortunately many of the most potent food motivators are bad. Take, for instance, using sweets as a reward. Birthday cake, containing sugar and saturated fat, celebrates a special day and becomes a lifelong ritual. Christmas, Easter, Valentine's Day—all use chocolate to convey love and holiday spirit. These are powerful images. In adulthood, have you ever unconsciously eaten a chocolate bar because you're a little down? The chocolate conjures up images of happier times. Eating it creates a feeling of comfort. Some of this good feeling is because chocolate contains neurotransmitters very much like endorphins that create a sense of well-being not long after you eat it.

There are two schools of thought on how to change one's diet. One holds that making gradual changes over time is the easiest, the least jarring, method. The other supports making a drastic change all at once so that reminders of old habits don't entice you back to your bad old ways. While I was in Cardiac Rehab, the prevailing view of the nutritionists I dealt with was to make the big changes. They reasoned that after a heart attack one's life was drastically changed anyway, so it would be easier to start with a new food regimen.

The "fresh start" approach was the choice I made. I knew that if I tried to wean myself off chocolate and cookies and all the other junk I sometimes ate, I would have relapses. Once I looked in the mirror and saw the bruises that blotched my face, it was easy to say, "You're not the person you were. All the old rules are gone. This is not a game you can cheat at and not get caught."

So, if we feel our food options shrinking, we need to get creative. Part of the objective is to fool our palates into thinking we're eating many of the things we have always eaten; their contents just shift.

Here's a good example of how to avoid dangerous fats yet still eat a favorite food. I have always loved Caesar salad: I love making it and I love eating it. However, this salad is a killer: eggs, Parmesan cheese, croutons cooked in butter. It was one of the first things to get excised from my menu.

However, after months went by, I missed my Caesar salad. By tinkering with how I made it, I found a way to give it a new, healthier incarnation. Now, instead of coddled eggs, I use Egg Beaters. Instead of generic vegetable oil, I use canola or olive oil. The croutons are now stir-fried in a wok using a lot of garlic and canola oil instead of butter. I still use Parmesan, but very sparingly, only for taste, filling in the rest of what I formerly used with fat-free Parmesan. Guess what? The salad tastes almost exactly the same as I always made it, but instead of being a heart-bomb, it's actually very healthy now. It's so good that guests frequently ask for the recipe.

The romaine lettuce provides one of the day's five-a-day vegetables or fruits (recommended by the USDA's Food and Nutrition Service); the canola oil provides the monounsaturated and polyunsaturated fat I need for energy, while also reducing LDLs and triglycerides; the Egg Beaters provide protein without cholesterol and saturated fat. There's nothing harmful in this salad. I need only to decide how much I'm going to have and if I should scale back on meat or fish for that day because, even though the fats in this salad are beneficial, too much will result in weight gain. I keep my fat intake to around forty grams per day, which works out to about 15 percent of my caloric intake. This is at the low end of what I am allowed, but I feel safer that way. Remember, you can have a healthy diet and have good blood values, but still gain weight.

In the short term, a few pounds up or down are not an issue. But if you begin a steady creep upward, look out. Your blood pressure will rise, increasing the risk of blood clots. If you already have plaque in your arteries, it's not a good idea to increase your clotting risk. And if you've already had a heart attack, extra weight makes your heart work more to pump fluids through a larger body. In the long term, weight gain cannot yield good effects.

One food danger I've found is with fat-free baked goods. Some fat-free brownies and cookies and pastries are very tasty, but to make them taste good without fat, the manufacturers add a lot of sugar. Sugar will raise triglyceride levels and can trigger small-particle LDL production. So I allow myself a little treat once in a while to offset my craving for chocolate, but I do not buy more than one container of whatever that treat is. If I have more in the house, I'm tempted to eat it. Here is one place where portion control is extremely important. Binge eating can offset weeks of progress.

Why do we crave fats so voraciously? Apart from the body's need for fat, fats taste good. Fat also triggers chemical receptors in the body that create a feeling of fullness and well-being. Quite literally, we feel better after eating fats. How many times have you fallen asleep after Thanksgiving dinner? It's the best nap of the year, isn't it? It's probably the largest intake of calories and fat of the year, too.

Guess what day the largest number of heart attacks occurs in the United States. Yes, it's on Thanksgiving, when even the heart-diseased break their diets and gorge. Dinner, dessert, then death.

Sorry, I don't like eating *that* much.

The American Heart Association suggests limiting one's intake of saturated fat to 7 percent of calories and total calories from fat to no more than 30 percent of one's diet. In an average two-hundred-pound, fairly active male, this would mean roughly 23 grams of saturated fat per day out of a total fat budget of 100 grams. In reality, the average American diet consists of much more saturated fat than 7 percent. One Big Mac supplies almost *all* the fat calories the average person needs for an entire day, and most of those calories are from saturated fats.

My approach sounds radical, but I avoid almost all saturated fats. Why consume any saturated fat you don't have to? If there are fat substitutes (poly- and monounsaturates) that have a beneficial effect on blood cholesterol levels, why consume saturated fats, which can only have a negative effect?

In my case, that means I don't use butter or whole milk or cream cheese or sour cream. I don't eat steak or french fries or prime rib. But guess what? Molly McButter sprinkled on food tastes just like butter. I fool my stomach with skim milk, fat-free cream cheese, and fat-free sour cream in recipes, and I barely notice the difference. No big sacrifice.

There is a weird twist in the American psyche that equates pleasure with being bad. If a food is particularly delicious or satisfying, it is called "decadent." We seem to take giggly enjoyment from "cheating" on our diets, as if in this dereliction we experience a wicked, smaller-scale version of big-time "cheating" such as at cards or on our spouses.

We indulge our pleasures of the flesh with the promise that we'll quit smoking tomorrow; we'll start exercising after the holidays; we'll make a New Year's resolution to cut drinking. Two weeks before vacation, we decide we need to look better in our bathing suits and we go on crash exercise-starvation regimens and land on the beach sore and weak. Are we nuts?

No, we're just human. We all do it. And we all regret it. The problem with carriers of heart-killer genes is that we have less leeway than our brethren. We have less time. We can make fewer mistakes because this gene works fast, slapping cholesterol onto our arteries and manipulating our blood chemistry.

Many people start their reforms in middle age, when their bodies can't keep up with the abuses they've heaped on them for three or four decades. Men feel the waning of sexual prowess and join health clubs to try to regain some of the verve of youth. Women feel their bodies sag and start aerobics and dye their hair.

But by middle age, those of us with the HeartStopper Effect could be dead. We don't have the luxury of reforming our lives after a couple of decades of even mild abuse. We can live a healthy, athletic lifestyle and still be struck down in our thirties and forties if we don't know we have a HeartStopper gene.

So, we have to be more vigilant about our lifestyles, and we have to be on some medical therapy. But this doesn't mean we have to live like monks. It's possible to retain the general form of our diets while making substitutions with many of the components. It's possible to have a drink now and then or to eat devil's food cake. It's just important to show moderation.

Imagine a thick, juicy steak. Baked potato with sour cream. A typical American dinner. Now imagine someone sprinkling arsenic all over the steak. Would you eat it? Yet the average American male will eat thousands of steaks over a lifetime, each one leaving behind a little arterial gift. For those of us with a killer gene, the steak might as well be poisoned.

Diet is important for everyone, but for carriers of a heart-killer gene, diet is *really* important. It's the difference between having liquid, unstable cholesterol plaque on one's arteries or having stabilized plaque. It does not take near-total blockage of a coronary artery to trigger a massive heart attack. All it takes is a tiny tear on the surface of the plaque, a little crack, just enough to get the blood clotting as it tries to repair what it perceives as a break in the artery itself.

Dietary habits are ingrained in us from childhood. They hang on tight. Each of us has a collection of specific foods we eat in specific ways. Think of an extreme example such as Thanksgiving. Some families use canned, jellied cranberry, the kind that makes a sucking sound as it slowly slides from the can. Others use the whole-berry sauce. Still others make their cranberry dish from scratch, using fresh, whole cranberries.

How many times has your family switched cranberry dishes? Can you imagine using the jellied cranberry one year, then the next year making fresh cranberry sauce? It would cause a revolt in the kitchen. Once a cranberry form is established in a family, it does not change.

Think about other foods and you will realize that there are all sorts of food rituals. How do you eat an Oreo cookie? Whole, or do you open it up and lick the filling first? How many Americans eat cereal in the morning because we ate it as kids, bombarded for years by a steady stream of Saturday-morning cartoon-show commercials?

Food habits are among the toughest to change. I've learned to trick myself. The secret is to substitute fat-free or low-fat alternatives for the foods one normally eats. Say you love hot dogs. They're loaded with fat. But did you know there are major-brand, fat-free hot dogs? With mustard and relish, the difference in taste is negligible.

Cutting down on fat does not mean going on a starvation diet. Almost all lunch meats now come in a fat-free form. You can still make a submarine sandwich that tastes as good as you remember, but with fat-free meats, fat-free mayonnaise, and olive or canola oil. I used these ingredients recently to make subs for guests without telling them what I was doing. After lunch they raved about the subs. Then I told them the ingredients. They were stunned. They also looked at me as if I had cheated them.

These new foods are out there. We just need to look for them.

Over the past two years, I've enjoyed the search for new foods. Maybe some of these products had been on the shelves before and I hadn't seen them, but suddenly I was finding fat-free cheeses and lunch meats and hot dogs and crackers. Yes, they did cost more than regular foods. Yes, some of them tasted bland, but by experimenting, I was able to find some good-tasting products that I worked into my diet. And when I compared the additional cost of these foods against what I was paying for prescriptions, it seemed meager. I've just viewed fat-free foods as another prescription I have to buy. The alternative is suffering and death. How could anyone put a price on avoiding that?

I've learned to cruise the aisles of my supermarket. I talk to the managers. I ask for things I don't see. Supermarket managers want to serve their customers. They don't mind ordering special items. This is their business. They love to talk about it. They want to find whatever small edge will keep customers coming to their store versus the one up the street.

I watched as my local supermarket added several items at my request. At first, I felt I was the only person buying the stuff, but over time I began to see items sold out as other shoppers discovered them. Then the shelf space of the fat-free items increased, always a sure indicator of sales. Obviously, others were buying these foods, too. Maybe they had been searching as well.

Now, just as I've introduced the option of healthy, fat-free and low-fat substitutes, I also need to warn against latching onto all fat-free foods and putting our brains on autopilot.

A widely believed myth, largely fostered by the processed-food industry, is that fat-free means okay to eat in vast quantities. If there's no fat, what's the problem?

Hundreds of foods are advertised as *cholesterol-free, low-fat, light,* or *fat-free.* This does not confer magical properties on these foods.

The problematic fat-free foods are desserts such as baked goods, ice cream, and frozen yogurt. We all have a weakness for these foods, whether they're brownies or cookies or hot fudge sundaes. When we see *fat-free* plastered all over the container, we're tempted to think we're home free. We're not. These foods in their normal state are butter, oil, flour, and sugar. When manufacturers decide to cut out the fat, they greatly increase sugar content to make the product tasty. It's fat and sugar that make most things taste good. Less of one requires more of the other.

Remember the definition of triglycerides? They are *fatty acids* used by the body as building blocks for other fat compounds. They increase rapidly with an increase in carbohydrate consumption, particularly simple carbohydrates such as sugar. So, eating fat-free ice cream or pastries may seem to be a way to avoid the fat trap, but in fact they can cause the same problem. Sugar gets made into triglycerides. Triglycerides get made into cholesterol. Even worse, if triglycerides increase to above 140 mg/dL, they trigger production of small-particle LDL, which starts to build up on artery walls.

Advertisers prey on the ignorance of the public. One of the biggest deceptions of the food industry is advertising that a food is *cholesterol-free* or *fat-free*. This is a meaningless claim if the food has a lot of sugar. It's just a back-door route to the same problem. While your body happily converts sugar to triglycerides to cholesterol or fat, you're proud of yourself for eating healthy food. Yet you couldn't be further from the truth. Read labels and don't let advertisers delude you into a false sense of security.

To be clear, I eat both fat-free foods and foods that contain fat in managing my total fat consumption. I may use fat-free deli meats for a sandwich at lunch. That is because I plan to have salmon for dinner. (The fat in salmon is largely monounsaturated.) I limit my fat-containing meat or fish to six ounces a day, but fat-free meats don't get counted as part of the six-ounce limit, so I use them to harmlessly satisfy my lunch-meat craving. If I'm going to use olive oil on a salad at dinner, I may use a fat-free salad dressing at lunch. I mix and match fat and fat-free to stay near my goal of keeping fat intake at 15 to 20 percent of my caloric intake. In this way I have made a drastic change in the fat type and content of what I eat, but I don't have to fight big battles with my long-ingrained food habits. And I'm starving my HeartStopper gene of the building blocks it needs to form small-particle LDL.

Since I'm on a low-fat diet, you might ask yourself why does the subtitle of this book warn of how a low-fat diet can kill you? Here's why. I eat fat-free foods to manage my total fat intake. My diet, though low in fat, particularly avoids saturated fats. What fats I do consume are either monounsaturated or polyunsaturated. These fats lower LDL and triglycerides rather than increase them as do saturated fats.

The standard approach of a low-fat, heart-healthy diet is to increase carbohydrate consumption. This is dangerous because carbohydrates are quickly turned into triglycerides, the basic building block needed by a HeartStopper gene to create unstable arterial plaque. If you don't know that your LDL subclass is type B, a low-fat diet can cause unstable arterial plaque and a heart attack.

In my diet, I have marginally increased protein intake to offset some of my fat reduction. The rest of my calories come from *complex* carbohydrates: fruits and vegetables, whole grain breads, oatmeal, brown rice, and nuts. Complex carbohydrates do not get digested as fast as simple carbohydrates; they do not normally cause a spike in triglycerides and LDL, unless one's fat consumption is very low.

My own experience has shown that when I was on an *extremely* low fat diet (5 percent of calories), my triglycerides and LDL *did* spike, even though I was eating complex carbohydrates. However, 5 percent of calories from fat is just too low; that level was bound to cause distortions in my blood chemistry. Also, I was not yet taking niacin, which counters LDL production and reverses the otherwise harmful effects of a low-fat diet for carriers of a HeartStopper gene.

So, if you dramatically cut fat consumption but a large portion of your fat budget is saturated fats, and if you then eat simple carbohydrates to make up those calories, you will continue to provide the building blocks necessary to create the HeartStopper Effect. Your body will continue to produce small-particle LDL. Even though you will feel a sense of accomplishment at the food sacrifices you are making, you will be doing nothing to improve your cardiac health. In fact, you will be accelerating growth of the unstable plaque that could kill you.

It is important to recognize that lowering fat intake will increase the likelihood that more carbohydrates will be converted to small-particle LDL and will contribute to unstable arterial plaque. To counteract this, carriers of HeartStopper genes should strictly limit saturated fat consumption, substituting mono- and polyunsaturated fats; should avoid sugar-rich foods such as candy, soft drinks, cake, cookies, pastries, and honey; and should at least be on niacin therapy. We have no choice but to eat carbohydrates, but we can prevent them from being harmful.

Here's a tool I developed to help manage my day-to-day fat consumption.

HOW TO CONSTRUCT YOUR PERSONAL FAT BUDGET

1. Your desired weight: _____ pounds.
2. Your daily calorie intake to achieve your desired weight.

Activity Level	Calories Needed per Pound per Day
Couch Potato	11
Moderately Active (exercise 2–3 times/week)	13
Active (exercise 4–5 times/week)	15
Very Active (exercise 6–7 times/week)	18

_____ x _____ = _____ Calories needed daily

Ideal weight   x   Activity level = Calories needed daily

Example: Target weight is 190 pounds for an Active individual.

190 x 15 = 2,850 calories needed daily

---

3. Determine your fat budget.

Fifteen to 30 percent of daily calories should come from fat, preferably mono- and polyunsaturated. Following are different levels of possible fat intake.

.15 x _____ = _____ ÷ 9 = Grams of fat

Calories needed daily   Calories

.20 x _____ = _____ ÷ 9 = Grams of fat

Calories needed daily   Calories

.25 x _____ = _____ ÷ 9 = Grams of fat

Calories needed daily   Calories

.30 x _____ = _____ ÷ 9 = Grams of fat

Calories needed daily   Calories

Example: .30 x 2,850 Calories needed daily ÷ 9 = 95 total fat grams daily

2,850 calories x .07 = 200 calories ÷ 9 = 22 grams of saturated fat daily

---

_____ **grams of fat per day is my personal fat budget**

Calories needed daily x .07 ÷ 9 = maximum grams of saturated fat per day

_____ **total allowable grams of saturated fat per day**

Now that we've established a fat budget, let's look at how to use this information.

The American Heart Association recommends that a diet not exceed 30 percent fat content with only 7 percent of that as saturated fat. I think this level is too high for me. I keep my dietary fat intake between 15 and 20 percent. However, for the sake of illustration, let's use a fat budget that's 28 percent of total calories (because the calculations are easier).

If one has a fat budget of 28 percent of total calories, then set aside 7 percent of that as the limit for saturated fat, leaving 21 percent available for mono- and polyunsaturated fats. An easy way to remember this is that for every gram of saturated fat you eat, you must eat three grams of unsaturated fat.

So, let's use an example. For lunch we have a sandwich made with a small chicken breast, as well as a salad on which we use canola oil and vinegar. The chicken breast contains six grams of saturated fat. To make this meal work, we need to eat eighteen grams of mono- or polyunsaturated fat. Bread may or may not contain saturated fat, depending on type, but for the sake of this example let's say the bread contains one gram of polyunsaturated fat per slice. That's two grams. A tablespoon of canola oil contains one gram of saturated fat, four grams of polyunsaturated fat, and eight grams of monounsaturated fat. Let's use three tablespoons of oil on the salad. Here's what our fat totals look like:

	Saturated Fat	Monounsaturated Fat	Polyunsaturated Fat
2 slices of oat bread			2 grams
1 chicken breast (6 oz)	6 grams		
3 tablespoons canola oil	3 grams	24 grams	12 grams
Totals	9 grams	24 grams	14 grams

Add monounsaturates and polyunsaturates (since both are beneficial) and we get the following:

Bad Fats	Good Fats
9 grams	38 grams

If we need three good fats for every bad fat, then for this meal we need at least 9 x 3 = 27 grams of good fat to counter the bad fat. In our example, we have 38 grams of good fat, so we have a very healthy meal in terms of fat balance. Remember, though, that the total fat consumption of this meal is 47 grams, a substantial portion of the average person's fat budget for the day.

Let's see how this meal fits into an active adult male's fat-budget calculations:

185 pounds x 14 calories per pound per day = 2,590 calories per day needed

2,590 calories per day x 28 percent = 725 calories from fat per day

725 ÷ 9 = 80 grams of fat allowed per day to maintain this body weight

2,590 calories x 7 percent = 181 ÷ 9 = 20 grams of saturated fat allowed out of the total of 80 grams per day

This means our subject could have a total of eighty grams of fat per day of which no more than twenty grams could be saturated fat and of which at least sixty grams should be unsaturated fats.

So, this meal has accounted for nine of the twenty grams of saturated fat allowed plus forty-seven of the sixty grams of mono- or polyunsaturated fats. Our subject could eat an additional eleven grams of saturated fat plus thirteen grams of mono- or polyunsaturated fat during the rest of the day to maintain a healthy balance of good fat/bad fat for the day.

My personal choice would be to eat no other saturated fats during the day and to use those eleven grams as mono- or polyunsaturated fats. I also don't have good luck trying to remember whether I have a carryover of good or bad fats from meal to meal. I find it easier to balance fats within each meal and then to forget about it.

I don't carry a laptop computer with me to make meal decisions. I keep a rough count of the number of fat grams I eat during the day. On any given day, I might wind up a few grams over or under my fat budget. However, I always make sure I err on the side of fewer saturated fats. I don't eat saturated fats unless there's not much choice. For instance, in olive oil, there are two grams of saturated fat per serving, but this is acceptable to me since there are also twelve grams of mono- and polyunsaturated fats in that same serving. The preponderance of the fats are good for me, so I don't worry about it. On the other hand, choosing saturated-fat-dripping spareribs off a restaurant menu is something I just wouldn't do.

To make these choices and the calculations needed to stay within a fat budget, let's examine how to use nutrition labeling. Here's a typical nutrition label I've made up for a cookie product. Notice that if a food contains fat, the label gives the total fat grams and then breaks this down into the different types of fats. This label shows only saturated fat, but if the food contained monounsaturated and polyunsaturated fats, you would see them listed, too. I typically will look for my good-fat/bad-fat ratio right here. I rarely eat a food that doesn't show at least three grams of good fat for every gram of bad fat because I worry too much that I'll forget if I eat something that's full of saturated fat and not balance it with something containing mostly unsaturated fat. But that's a matter of choice.

Nutrition Facts		
Imaginary Cookies		
Serving Size 10 cookies		
Servings Per Container 5		
Amount Per Serving		
Calories 120		
Calories from Fat 25		
		% Daily Value
Total Fat 2.5g		4%
Saturated Fat 0g		0%
Cholesterol 0mg		0%
Sodium 90mg		4%
Total Carbohydrate 23g		8%
Dietary Fiber 1g		4%
Sugars 4g		
Protein 2g		

With most food labels, if you add all the fats listed, they don't always equal the total fat amount. In this example you see total fats of 2.5 grams, but saturated fats as zero. What are the other fats? I refer to these unnamed fats as phantom fats. If you check the ingredient list that usually appears under a nutrition label, you'll find that a food that has these unitemized phantom fats frequently contains "hydrogenated soybean or cottonseed oil," particularly if it is a baked good. Manufacturers use these oils because they are cheap. These oils contain trans-fatty acids that act very much like saturated fats. Recent research suggests that the arterial effects of trans-fatty acids are even worse than saturated fats. In this example, it would be easy to think one was buying a perfectly safe product that contained no saturated fats. Technically, because they are not saturated fats, the manufacturer doesn't have to list trans-fatty acids, but it's a sneaky way to sidestep the issue to save a few pennies.

To be safe, I add up phantom fats with the saturated fats. So, if a food's total fat content shows a majority of saturated fats and phantom fats, I don't eat it. In the example label, if the ingredient list showed the fat source as hydrogenated soybean oil, I wouldn't buy the product.

However, let's say the fat source listed as an ingredient was canola oil, which is over 90 percent mono- and polyunsaturated fats. Then the phantom fats would be good fats. Then the 2.5 grams of fat in this label would be primarily mono- and polyunsaturated. This would be a good product for anyone, but particularly for someone with the HeartStopper Effect. The saturated fat content of canola oil in a serving would be less than .25 gram and it would be listed as zero as shown. (Anything under .5 grams is listed as zero.) So, when the total fats don't equal the fats listed, assume phantom fats and look at the ingredient list for clarification. If you have trouble identifying the fat source, assume it is a trans-fatty acid, add it to the saturated fat, and if the phantom fats and saturated fats total more than 25 percent of the fat content, don't buy the product.

It's also important to look at the lines on labels that identify sugars, particularly when examining fat-free foods. Don't get suckered by the banner across the package front that screams FAT-FREE. Recent articles I've read show that people usually eat double to triple their normal servings of foods that are fat-free because they think they have died and gone to heaven; they don't have to worry about fat content.

Remember that our bodies will make fat out of sugar. Eating sugar or fat has the same result: triglycerides will jump and then LDLs will rise. This wouldn't be good for a regular heart patient, but if you have the HeartStopper Effect, it's even worse; your body will then produce the dangerous small-particle LDL.

The label on the following page is from a package of a nationally known brand of fat-free chocolate cupcakes. Hurrah, there's no fat. We should dive in, right? But look at that sugar content: thirty-three grams of sugar per serving! Thirty-three grams of sugar is *eleven* teaspoons. Imagine a cup of coffee with eleven teaspoons of sugar in it. You'd think someone who drank it was nuts. So why might that be okay in a cupcake? And a serving is one cupcake. Do you really think you'll eat only one cupcake?

I've tried these cupcakes. They're very good. I bought them when I was in a hurry and I thought the label said three grams of sugar per serving. I took them home and ate one with a cold glass of milk. I was suddenly a child again. I swear, I went into a sugar high. After all the months of restricting my diet, all the chocolate longings were suddenly relieved. I had found the Holy Grail, a delicious fat-free dessert that was also low in sugar. The damn thing was so good, I ate two more.

Nutrition Facts	
Chocolate Cupcakes	
Serving Size 1 cupcake	
Servings Per Container 4	
Amount Per Serving	
Calories 160	
Calories from Fat 0	
	% Daily Value
Total Fat 0g	**0%**
Saturated Fat 0g	**0%**
Cholesterol 0mg	**0%**
Sodium 160mg	**6%**
Total Carbohydrate 39g	**13%**
Dietary Fiber 2g	**8%**
Sugars 33g	
Protein 1g	

Then I reread the label and thought I was seeing things. I realized my mistake and a chill ran through me. When I saw that, instead of eating nine grams of sugar as I'd thought, I'd eaten ninety-nine grams (thirty-three teaspoons) of sugar in five minutes, I almost had a heart attack from realizing how stupid I was. For the rest of that day I kept checking my pocket to make sure I had my nitroglycerin pills. I was sure I would need them.

I no longer go near my supermarket's cupcake display. The temptation is too great and my eyesight is too poor.

FOOD GUIDE PYRAMID

This is the USDA Food Guide Pyramid that appears on many food packages. It shows the various food groups and recommended numbers of servings of each per day. Notice, at the pyramid's broad base are carbohydrates. Most diets recommend that breads, cereals, rice, and pasta should be the mainstay of one's food intake. Low-fat diets substitute calories normally eaten as fat with foods from this group. For most people, this is good advice. However, for people with the HeartStopper Effect, this is

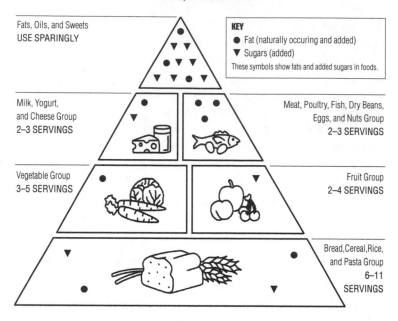

Fats, Oils, and Sweets
USE SPARINGLY

KEY
● Fat (naturally occuring and added)
▼ Sugars (added)
These symbols show fats and added sugars in foods.

Milk, Yogurt,
and Cheese Group
2–3 SERVINGS

Meat, Poultry, Fish, Dry Beans,
Eggs, and Nuts Group
2–3 SERVINGS

Vegetable Group
3–5 SERVINGS

Fruit Group
2–4 SERVINGS

Bread, Cereal, Rice,
and Pasta Group
6–11
SERVINGS

dangerous because the genetic mutations that cause the Heart-Stopper Effect will use added carbohydrates to make simple sugars that will increase triglycerides and trigger the production of dangerous small-particle LDL. For this reason, drug therapy is essential to combat the naturally destructive effects and to allow one to eat carbohydrates safely.

FOOD AND FAT GUIDE

I've explained why it's important to shift from bad-fat consumption to good-fat consumption, and I've shown you how to budget the amount of fat you should have in your diet. So, what do you do with this information? On the following page are basic food groups from which you can choose. In general, select foods from the Low Fat and Medium Fat columns and you'll be able to eat more food and stay within your fat budget. However, you need to consult the food labels on specific foods to see the exact fat content per serving and the amount of mono- and polyunsaturated fats versus saturated fat. In the previous section, I showed you how to interpret these labels.

A simple rule of thumb is to cut out pastries, cakes, candy, cookies, and sweet drinks. Eat whole-grain foods, vegetables, fruits, lean poultry, and fish. Avoid beef, pork, lamb, and duck.

I have marked particular foods with a small heart ♥. These are foods that may appear in the High Fat or Very High Fat columns, but they contain good fats—monounsaturated and polyunsaturated fats. As you calculate portions within your fat budget, make sure to include some of these foods, but be sure you don't exceed your budget.

DAIRY GROUP

Low Fat: <15%	Medium Fat:15–30%	High Fat: 30–50%	Very High Fat: >50%
Skim milk	1 percent milk	2 percent milk	Whole milk
Dry-curd cottage cheese	Low-fat cottage cheese (sodium)	Creamed cottage cheese (sodium)	
Nonfat yogurt	Plain low-fat yogurt		
Fruit-flavored nonfat yogurt (sugar)	Fruit-flavored low-fat yogurt (sugar) Plain low-fat yogurt		
Nonfat frozen yogurt (sugar)	Low-fat frozen yogurt (sugar) Ice milk (sugar)	Regular ice cream	Gourmet ice cream
			Nondairy creamers
			Cream, sour cream, half & half, butter
		Reduced-calorie cheeses (sodium)	Most cheeses

Most frozen yogurts, ice milk, and ice cream are high in sugar, even though they may be nonfat or low-fat. Some brands now use artificial sweeteners and are advertised as "sugar-free."

FRUITS AND VEGETABLES

Low Fat: <15%	Medium Fat: 15–30%	High Fat: 30–50%	Very High Fat: >50%
Plain vegetables with no added sauces; fresh or frozen, or canned		French fries Hash browns	♥ Avocados ♥ Olives (sodium) Coconut, Coconut Milk Onion rings (fried)
Fruits; fresh, frozen, canned (sugar) or dried (sugar)			

Any processed fruits and vegetables may contain added salt, sugar, or fat. Check the package labels.

GRAINS AND CEREAL FOODS

Low Fat: <15%	Medium Fat: 15–30%	High Fat: 30–50%	Very High Fat: >50%
Flour made from wheat, corn, barley, rice, rye, and bulgur Most breads Some breakfast cereals Bagels Pita bread Corn tortillas Grits Noodles and pasta Popcorn (air-popped) Rice cakes Ry-Krisp Pretzels (sodium)	Corn bread from mix Flour tortillas ♥ Oatmeal Rolls and buns Wheat germ Some crackers	Muffins Granola Popcorn (popped in oil) Taco shells Most snack crackers Biscuits	Potato and other chips Croissants Pastries

Popcorn and muffins, though high in fat, could be made with canola oil and thus could be beneficial if you stay within your fat budget.

FISH

Low Fat: <15%	Medium Fat: 15–30%	High Fat: 30–50%	Very High Fat: >50%
Cod, flounder, haddock, halibut, perch, sea bass, sole, abalone, crayfish, scallops, shrimp Canned tuna (in water) Octopus Squid (cholesterol)	Bass, catfish, smelts, sturgeon, clams, crab, mussels, oysters Fresh tuna Lobster	♥ Albacore tuna Carp ♥ Salmon Canned tuna (in oil, drained)	♥ Anchovies ♥ Herring ♥ Mackerel ♥ Trout Sardines (cholesterol) Shad Eel Canned tuna (in oil)

Fish contain beneficial oils known as omega-3 fatty acids.
Canned, dried, and pickled fish usually have high sodium content.

POULTRY

Low Fat: <15%	Medium Fat: 15–30%	High Fat: 30–50%	Very High Fat: >50%
Egg whites	Chicken and turkey; light meat without skin Turkey-breast lunch meats	Chicken and turkey; light meat with skin Chicken and turkey; dark meat without skin Duck and goose without skin Turkey lunch meats (sodium)	Chicken and turkey; dark meat with skin Duck and goose with skin Egg yolks (cholesterol) Whole eggs (cholesterol) Ground turkey

Many lunch meats are now available in nonfat form and provide needed protein, but have no impact on your fat budget.

MEATS

Low Fat: <15%	Medium Fat: 15–30%	High Fat: 30–50%	Very High Fat: >50%

	Trimmed:
	  Beef (flank,
	    round, or tips)
	  Pork tenderloin
	  Veal (loin, round,
	    or shoulder)
	  Liver (cholesterol)
	  Low-fat lunch meats
	    (less than 2 grams
	    of fat per ounce)
		Trimmed:
		  Beef or veal
		  Fresh ham
		  Cured ham
		    (sodium)
		  Kidneys
		    (cholesterol)
		  Heart (cholesterol)
		  Canadian Bacon
		    (sodium)
			Partially trimmed:
			  Beef, veal, lamb,
			    pork
			  Bacon or sausage
			    (sodium)
			  Lunch meats
			    (sodium)
			  Hot dogs (sodium)
			  Brains (cholesterol)
			  Tongue (cholesterol)

No meats are high in poly- or monounsaturated fats.

NUTS AND LEGUMES

Low Fat: <15%	Medium Fat: 15–30%	High Fat: 30–50%	Very High Fat: >50%

Dried beans
Dried peas
Lentils
Chestnuts
		♥ Soybeans
		♥ Tofu
			♥ Most nuts and
			    seeds
			♥ Peanuts and
			    peanut butter
			  Cashews
			  Macadamia nuts
			  Brazil nuts

Canned and packaged nuts usually contain high amounts of added sodium.

PACKAGED AND FAST FOODS

Low Fat: <15%	Medium Fat:15–30%	High Fat: 30–50%	Very High Fat: >50%
Spaghetti with tomato sauce Bouillons Broth Consomme	Some diet TV dinners Some canned stews Vegetarian baked beans Some cheese pizzas Most soups Vegetarian refried beans	Fish sticks Fish sandwich Chili with beans Burrito, refried beans Cheeseburger, hamburger Spaghetti with meat sauce Macaroni and cheese Taco, tostada French fries	Chili con carne Fried chicken Hot dogs Falafel Fried pork rinds Snack chips Nachos Cheddar-cheese soup Most cream soups

CONDIMENTS

Low Fat: <15%	Medium Fat: 15–30%	High Fat: 30–50%	Very High Fat: >50%
Spices Vinegar Horseradish Tabasco sauce Salt Soy sauce Mustard Chili sauce Ketchup Pickles & relish No-oil salad dressings			Mayonnaise Salad dressings with oil or creamy dressings

DESSERTS

Low Fat: <15%	Medium Fat: 15–30%	High Fat: 30–50%	Very High Fat: >50%

Sugar
Honey
Molasses
Syrups
Jellies & jams
Angel food cake
Fig bars
Hard candies
Mints
Marshmallows
Gelatin desserts
Sherbets
Pudding made
  from skim milk
Fruit ices
Soft drinks
Frozen nonfat
  yogurt
	Animal crackers
	Ginger snaps
	Graham crackers
	Ice milk
	Pudding
	Frozen low-fat
	  yogurt
	Cocoa powder
		Cakes
		Cookies
		Granola bars
		Doughnuts
		Pastries
		Pies
		Candy bars
		Regular ice cream
		Custards
		Tofu frozen desserts
			Chocolate in all its
			  forms
			Gourmet ice cream

CHAPTER 18

Exercise

A year after my heart attack, I needed to have my gallbladder removed due to developing gallstones. (This was a side effect of a medication I was trying.) After surgery, I could not exercise for several weeks. I felt tired all the time, but I was eager to get back to it. As soon as my doctor said I could start exercising again, I did. It took me two weeks of sweaty, hard work to approach my previous activity levels. My physical and emotional improvement was dramatic. I felt better, slept better, and was in much better spirits.

Here are the lessons I've learned. First, I never push myself too far. We Americans tend to do everything to excess. When we start an exercise regimen, we go nuts. Within days we are so sore we stop exercising.

The slow approach I originally took to build up my heart was forced on me. I was not able to overdo it. I started out on the treadmill in rehab at .7 miles per hour and slowly built up to 3.5 miles per hour with three degrees of incline. This took four months. Not until I had this aerobic base did I begin adding some muscle-toning exercises. This slow approach kept me from backsliding.

There's a great machine at my health club called a Gravitron, made by StairMaster. It's designed for pull-ups and dips and gives a great workout to the upper body. What I really like is that it adjusts your effective body weight through a hydraulic system that supports the small platform on which you stand. I can work out at my full body weight or any percentage of it.

This is an excellent machine for someone who has cardiac damage because it allows for a perfect combination of factors: light weights and many repetitions. It's also great for women to build upper-body strength without struggling with free weights. I routinely work out at about 30 percent of my body weight.

Yes, the heavy lifters look at me as if I'm some kind of pansy. But my regimen is not designed for muscle mass. Its goal is a healthy heart, good muscle tone, and no excess weight. Cardiac patients should not use heavy weights for exercise. When muscles strain, blood pressure in the body surges momentarily to levels far above normal. Even if you are on a pressure-lowering medication, heavy lifting will cause spikes in your average blood pressure.

This is dangerous because surges in blood pressure can cause stretching in the scar tissue created by a heart attack. As this tissue stretches, the heart gets larger and less efficient. If the heart gets too big, it can't pump with sufficient pressure to move fluids through the body. The result is congestive heart failure. The lungs slowly fill with fluid and the patient literally drowns.

If you are post–heart attack, forget about pumping iron. The price of achieving a Schwarzeneggerian physique will be heart damage. It's not better to look good than to feel good, dahling.

There's one other factor to consider if you're obsessed with bulking up. The more weight you put on, whether muscle or fat, the higher your blood pressure will usually go. It's better to be at the lower end of your individual weight range than the high end. If you're taking a blood-pressure-lowering medication, you will need more of it if you weigh more. The more medicine one takes, the greater are the side effects: possible dizziness, fatigue, drowsiness, and—oh, yes—impotence. Of course, the choice is yours, men, but it hardly seems worthwhile to spend long hours power-lifting to become more physically attractive if you can't then deliver.

In general, I'm most comfortable using machines that target specific muscle groups, but the same results can be achieved with free weights. I like the machines because I can set them specifically for the performance level I want. But that's just personal preference.

The ideal cardiac workout involves aerobic activity such as treadmill, stationary bike, stair-stepper, Nordic Track, or any other repetitive activity you can maintain for thirty to forty minutes to raise your heart rate. Aerobics should then be followed by light weight training or circuit training. The aerobics keep the heart in shape; the weights tone the other muscles.

My personal exercise target is forty minutes of treadmill to get my pulse between 80 and 100 beats per minute. This is a departure from the calculations you normally see for aerobic heart rates. At my age, the charts say I should reach a level of 140 to 150 beats per minute. However, that's the recommendation for a healthy, undamaged heart. In my case, such a rate would not be beneficial.

Make sure you consult your doctor for the target range best for you. It will vary depending on your age, condition, and the amount of arterial blockage or damage to your heart.

Another key factor is whether you are on a beta-blocker or ACE inhibitor. These drugs slow the heart rate, much like a governor on a car engine. It's literally impossible for me to achieve 150 beats per minute. I struggle to get to 100.

I had to get away from the idea that more was better. It's not necessary to come back from the gym like a wet dish towel. My total workout takes fifty to sixty minutes three or four times a week.

A few years ago, I would have laughed if anyone suggested joining a health club. The idea of paying for exercise seemed ludicrous when all I had to do was step out my front door to get all the exercise I could ever want. Every day I took my dog for long walks. I did push-ups and sit-ups and stomach crunches and stretching. I was in great shape and it was free. But after my heart attack, I had problems with outdoor exercise.

I'm now more sensitive to heat and cold. When the weather is extreme in summer or winter, I am less likely to exercise. If there's a snowstorm or it's raining or the temperature is over a hundred, one has the perfect excuse not to exercise. The problem is that it can be foul outside several days in a row. Once you break routine, it's so easy to be lazy. The result is dangerous. The air-conditioned stasis of the health club makes every day's environment optimal.

There's a more pointed factor, as well. When it's cold outside, the human body constricts exterior blood vessels to retain heat. Constricted blood vessels raise blood pressure, a no-no. Conversely, hot weather causes blood vessels to expand as the body tries to shed excess heat. This lowers blood pressure. If it's too hot outside, one risks light-headedness and even fainting.

Humidity is also a big factor. High humidity stresses the heart. In high humidity, the body has to work harder to keep a steady temperature because sweat doesn't evaporate as well as in low humidity.

My cardiologist suggested a simple formula to determine if I should walk or take light exercise outdoors. It's called the 150-degree rule. Add the temperature (in Fahrenheit) to the relative humidity. If they total more than 150, it's not good to exercise outdoors. Under 150 is okay. So, for example, it's a sunny day with a temperature of 70 and a relative humidity of 60 percent. Add them for a total index of 130. It's a good day for outdoor exercise.

Now, there are exceptions. In Southwest cities such as Phoenix or Las Vegas, the temperature could be 110 with only 10 percent humidity. The total of the two figures is 120, but exercising in 110 degrees is not a good idea for anyone, not to mention heart patients.

In a place like Washington, D.C., which gets very humid in the summer, it's not unlikely to have a day where the relative humidity is 90 percent and the temperature is 75 degrees. It doesn't *feel* that hot, but if you add the temperature and humidity, you see a total of 165. Ten minutes into a run, you'd be panting like a dog in a hot car. Use common sense.

I always thought exercising indoors would be boring. I used to think that nothing could be worse than walking in place on a treadmill. How my opinions have changed. I now like the treadmill more than any other piece of equipment. It gives me forty minutes of uninterrupted thinking. It's almost like meditation. (I mentally composed most of this book on a treadmill.)

If anyone still needs convincing on the need for exercise, there's one other little-known benefit. Exercise improves blood chemistry by raising HDL. Just twenty minutes of aerobic exercise a day can have a significant effect on the cholesterol/HDL ratio and lower overall cardiac risk. Conversely, no exercise lowers HDL and increases risk.

Just to give you a point of reference, here's my exercise regimen, performed three or four times per week. All of this takes less than an hour.

Warm-up stretching:	5 minutes
Treadmill:	40 minutes or 2 miles
Gravitron:	30 dips and 30 pull-ups at 30 percent body weight
Stomach crunches:	35 repetitions
Biceps machine:	10–15 repetitions
Triceps machine:	10–15 repetitions

MEASURING HEART RATE

Earlier I mentioned achieving a target heart rate during aerobic exercise. How does one measure this? There are several ways.

First, some exercise machines are fitted with heart-monitoring equipment. One type of exercise bike, for example, has sensors in the handlebars that constantly track heart rate and display it on the instrument screen. Some sophisticated treadmills and stair-steppers have a heart monitor that straps around the chest. The machine actually adjusts its exercise difficulty to match the target heart rate you program into the machine. Other treadmills have you enter the number of heartbeats you have in a ten-second interval and then they calculate your heart rate.

I use my wristwatch, which has a second hand. Not very sophisticated, but it works.

The most difficult part of manually measuring your pulse is finding it! Forget about wrists. The easiest way to measure heartbeats is to press the tips of your fingers into the major blood vessels in your neck. Feel under your ear for the point where your jawbone ends. Then feel down your jawbone to the right angle where the bone aims forward. Under that point, press your fingers into the soft part of your neck. Don't be afraid, you won't hurt yourself. You should feel a strong pulse. (It doesn't matter which side of your neck you use.)

Using a second timer, measure fifteen seconds as you count

your heartbeats. Multiply your count by four. That's your heart rate. For example, if you counted twenty-two beats, your rate is eighty-eight beats per minute. It takes a little practice, but it's important information to get the most out of your aerobic workout.

You may find that the vibrations from your exercise make it difficult to feel your pulse. Just step off the treadmill or stop whatever you're doing for the fifteen seconds it takes to measure. Then start right up again.

I've described what I do to stay fit. You may need a different regimen. But the crux of the matter is that you need regular aerobic exercise. Take your spouse for a walk in the evening—swim, ride a bike, but do *something*.

Remember at the beginning of the previous chapter I said that the most important word in being healthy is *consistency?* It is the difference between feeling sickly and feeling energetic. It's the difference between staying out of the hospital and a ride in an ambulance. It will add pleasurable years to your life.

BODY MASS INDEX

Here's a great way to quickly see if you need more exercise. Body mass index (BMI) is a good general indicator of one's health and of one's potential for coronary problems. BMI is an index that compares weight to size. In general, the higher one's BMI, the more fat one is carrying. The lower the number, the more healthy one is. There are exceptions. Because of muscle's greater density than fat, a bodybuilder could have a high BMI yet low body fat. But in general, BMI is a quick way to see if you need to shed some pounds.

To find your BMI, multiply your weight in pounds by 703, then divide by your height in inches squared. A healthy BMI is twenty-four or less.

> Example: I am 6'2" and weigh 185 pounds.
> 185 pounds x 703 = 130,055
> 6'2" = 74 inches
> 74" x 74" = 5,476
> 130,055 ÷ 5,476 = 23.75 BMI

Exercise

Look up my height in the left-hand column of the chart below. Then read across the row and find my weight or the closest number to it (in this case 187). It is in the BMI column marked 24. Look up and see that this column is marked "Healthy." Look at the next column to the right. If I gained eight pounds, I would be considered overweight.

You can save doing the calculations by finding the row that shows your height and reading across until you find the weight closest to yours.

BODY MASS INDEX

	Healthy	Healthy	Moderately Overweight	Overweight	Overweight	Very Overweight
BMI >>	23	24	25	26	27	28
5'	118	123	128	133	138	143
5'1"	122	127	132	137	143	148
5'3"	130	135	141	146	152	158
5'5"	138	144	150	156	162	168
5'7"	146	153	159	166	172	178
5'9"	155	162	169	176	182	189
5'11"	165	172	179	186	193	200
6'1"	174	182	189	197	204	212
6'2"	179	187	195	202	210	218
6'3"	184	192	200	208	216	224

To calculate your own BMI, fill in the blanks:

A. Your weight in pounds: _____ x 703 = _____

B. Your height in inches: _____ x your height in inches = _____

Divide the result of A by the result of B. The result is _____, your body mass index.

Compare your BMI to the chart. If your BMI is 25 or above, you need to lose weight.

If you have ever tracked your BMI before, you may note that your old chart says you are in the healthy category, but the above chart says you are overweight. This is because the National Heart, Lungs, and Blood Institute (part of the National Institutes of Health) made the BMI calculation more stringent and issued a new index in 1998. The BMI columns marked 25 and 26 were previously marked healthy, but are now considered overweight. So, if you were at the margin, suddenly overnight you lost the option to eat cheesecake.

CHAPTER 19

Stress Reduction

Night is a fearful time for me. There is not a night that I don't go to bed wondering if I will see the dawn. No matter how tired I am, I still feel a ripple of fear course through me as I approach sleep. To me the unconsciousness of sleep is not far from the void I found myself in when my heart arrested.

Some anomaly in my biological clock causes me to wake up in the middle of the night. It creates an ominous moment for me. Sometimes it is a dream that pulls me to the surface of consciousness. Sometimes it is nothing more than the furnace switching on. But in that first bleary moment of waking, I remember how I woke in the middle of the night to fight off death on May 9, 1996.

On waking, I perform a mental check much like a pilot readying for takeoff. Do I have chest pain? How am I breathing? Any small muscular ache becomes a point of focus. Is the pain deep inside? Is it nothing more than the result of exercise—a pulled stomach muscle, a sore back?

It is in what Ingmar Bergman called the hour of the wolf—the hour before dawn when life is at an ebb and when most deaths occur—that I lie back and catalog the many twinges and throbs that go unnoticed during the day. I feel my pulse. Is it steady? Strong or weak?

I avoid until last the insistent throbbing in the center of my chest. Yes, again I have them. PVCs, short for premature ventricular contractions. In a normal heart, the four chambers of the heart contract in a regular sequence that moves blood as efficiently as possible. In through the right atrium, out through the right ventricle to the lungs, then back into the heart through the left atrium and out via the left ventricle. It is the left ventricle that gives the blood its final push back into the body.

For post-heart-attack patients who have cardiac damage, there is usually a change in the way the heart pumps. Just look at an electrocardiogram before and after the attack. The lines that mark the electrical nerve impulses that fire the heart's contractions are different. The electrical wiring has changed. And so has the way the heart pumps.

In my case, the damage is in the left ventricle. Because of the damage, this part of the heart sometimes gets its electrical signals crossed and its fibers contract at the wrong time, usually ahead of schedule. This is called premature ventricular contraction. When it happens, the left ventricle squeezes before the rest of the heart is ready, and an inefficient pump occurs. Some blood may be backed into the heart, and the outflow during that beat is less than normal.

Other parts of the heart can occasionally fire prematurely. Next most likely is the atrium. When this occurs, it's called premature atrial contraction (PAC).

How serious is a PAC or PVC? One is insignificant. Hundreds are considered minor. In fact, in a normal human, it is common to have several thousand PVCs a day. We don't usually even notice them. But heart patients tend to notice anything irregular about what suddenly becomes the most important organ in the body.

At 4 A.M., I can feel the out-of-sync thumping in my chest. It feels like a tiny fist is hammering against my rib cage. I change position and sometimes it stops. Sometimes I get up and move around, trying to provide a different set of stimuli to change the way my heart is performing.

Usually, the PVCs pass in a few minutes. But sometimes they go on intermittently for hours. For weeks after I got out of the hospital following my heart attack, I had to sleep propped up with three big cushions behind me to stop the PVCs. Gradually, as weeks went by, I was able to reduce the number of pillows until I could once again sleep flat.

What causes them? I have gathered a personal encyclopedia of stimuli that I try to avoid to keep the PVCs at bay. If I eat too much, the pressure within my body cavity seems to bring on PVCs. If I lie in certain positions, usually on my left side, sometimes on my stomach, this can bring them on. Allergies and head-cold remedies can cause PVCs. Also, caffeine and other stimulants cause PVCs and should generally be avoided.

Sometimes when the weather is cold and I feel shivery, I can feel the tiny warning. Particularly when I get stressed, such as when someone cuts me off in traffic, again the little fist reminds me of my vulnerability.

It reminds me of the servants who ran behind the chariots of the Roman emperors of old. When the chariot stopped, the job of each servant was to occasionally whisper in the ear of his master, "Those whom the gods would destroy, they first praise. Glory is fleeting." It was a grim reminder that no matter how much glory was heaped on the head of a caesar, it was not under caesar's control and could disappear just as quickly as it had arrived.

I envision my reminder with his little fist inside my chest. Whenever I become too happy or start feeling as vigorous as I did before my heart attack, this little troll pounds his fist into me and says, "Your days are numbered. How do you want to spend them?"

I can rail about the idiots in traffic or I can look out the window at the stark, distant beauty of the Sierra Nevada. I can fume about standing in line at the post office or I can admire the colorful stamps in the display case and think about which stamps would be most appropriate to send to various people I know. I can rant about the early darkness of the winter evenings or I can take my telescope out on the deck and show my daughter the moons of Jupiter.

We all talk about reducing stress. Hundreds of books and therapy programs are designed to reduce the pressures of daily life. How long do we change our behavior after reading one of these books or attending one of these classes? A week? Maybe a few months? But then the boss does something capricious and stupid and we have to work overtime, or one of the kids puts a dent in the new car. The old familiar emotions kick in and blood pressure rises and the seething begins.

It's modern life. We all deal with stress, but it's crucial for the heart patient to do it effectively. Stress is one of the four pillars that must be mastered to have optimum cardiac health. The others are diet, exercise, and medication.

What changes have I made in my life to reduce stress, to try to be calmer? Let's start with the most basic concepts.

We cannot change other people, we cannot control our environment. We can only change ourselves. Accepting this is the only way to get control of stress. Stress does not come from outside the body; it comes from within.

How can I say this? The jerk who flipped me the finger as he made a right turn in front of me from the left lane is at fault, right? He's the reason the adrenaline pumped into my system; he's the reason I'm angry. Right?

Wrong. I can scream at him from the confines of my car and damn his lineage, but I cannot prevent him from doing it to someone else any more than I could have prevented him from cutting in front of me. Is that not the real source of my anger? I could not make him do what I thought was right; I can't hold him accountable for his dangerous actions. He won't do what I want.

Is this not the source of most anger? What, after all, is the bottom line of most arguments? The person I'm arguing with just doesn't see my point of view. If he did, he'd realize he was wrong and he'd agree with me. Right?

If we think back over our lives, how many times have we seen one party in an argument suddenly say to the other, "Gee, you're right. I don't know how I could have thought what I thought. I can't believe the error of my ways. I agree with you completely."

I have *never* seen this happen. The combatants often go on to a fistfight, a divorce, or they just never speak to each other again. In the political arena, rather than admit to being wrong, world leaders go to war. All in the name of being *right*.

So, if the experience of life has shown that it is the rarest of occurrences for someone to suddenly change his mind, why not accept that as reality and model our responses to that fact? This would have been a heretical thought when I was twenty, when I was happy to debate anyone on any subject for as long as it took to win. But now, at forty-eight, with a heart attack behind me, what price must I pay for being right? How valuable to me is it to be *dead* right?

So now, during rush hour, I *expect* someone to do something dangerous and stupid. I expect to be cut off, tailgated, and generally abused by some kamikaze commuter in a sport utility vehicle. If I expect these things and they happen, I can take satisfaction in being a genius at prediction. However, I'm no longer concerned with making the other guy see that he's wrong or with retaliating against him. In thirty seconds, the Neanderthal driver is off my radar screen as I think about something productive for me.

I choose to withdraw from the senseless hurly-burly. I choose to focus on my family and my internal life. I am controlling what I can control and not worrying about the rest.

Easy to say, but how to do it?

There are numerous techniques to get started. For instance, yoga and meditation work well for some people. For others, retreating into a favorite room to listen to music offers solace. Or reading a book on the back porch might be the ticket. The idea is to get to a quiet place in the mind so that one understands that the option of calmness exists.

But what about in traffic? At the store? At work?

When I was in Cardiac Rehab, in addition to exercise and nutrition training, I also had training in yoga and meditation three times a week. Though I was skeptical about this when I first started, it did not take long for me to realize that yoga and meditation offered powerful methods for controlling stress. I learned one important technique that is the foundation to maintaining my calm. Try this. Find a quiet place and sit down in a comfortable position. The place could be your bedroom, under a tree, anywhere you find peaceful and comfortable. Now close your eyes and think of nothing. As thoughts try to get your attention, recognize that they're there, but don't pursue them.

Thinking of nothing is incredibly difficult. As soon as you try, it seems your brain perversely tries to fill you with things you need to do, things you forgot, just anything to distract you. The first time you try this, it will be difficult. Set the limited goal of trying to clear your mind for five minutes. Inhale deeply, preferably through your nose, and exhale deeply so that you totally empty your lungs. When you inhale, push outward with the muscles of your belly to allow all the air possible to flow into you. When you exhale, contract the stomach muscles first to drive the air out of your lower body first, then your upper lungs, until you are empty. This technique is derived from yoga and is effective at relaxing the body so the mind can follow.

Do this several days in a row. Then, when you have had some modest success in relaxation breathing and in keeping calm, introduce another element. Think of some particular place, sensation, sound, or person that is pleasing to you. (To learn this technique, I used a photograph of my wife in which she has a beaming smile.) Think of this thought target to the exclusion of all else. This should be easier than trying to think of nothing, because with something in your focus, it's not difficult to push off other thoughts as they approach.

Focus on your thought target for five minutes while you perform the relaxation breathing. At first, this may seem like a long time. As you become more skilled in the technique, the time will fly past. You will be able to spend ten, then twenty minutes in this state without difficulty.

It may be easier to do this if you are reclined, but the danger is that you will fall asleep. Falling asleep is wonderful, but it negates the aspect of being able to reduce your stress wherever you are, so I suggest you sit up. You can't just fall asleep at work or while driving.

Eventually, when this relaxation technique becomes easy for you, you will be able to perform it anywhere. If you are feeling stressed at the office, you can take a short break and refocus yourself.

One day while I was driving, I noticed I felt particularly peaceful and happy. The air conditioner was soughing quietly and my whole body was bathed in cool air. The stream from one vent kept tugging at my hair. I found myself saying the word *cool* in my mind. *Cooool*. It was as if the word and the sensation were one and the same. I said it over and over. *Cooool.* The image and the sensation set themselves in my brain.

Now whenever I feel rushed, my foot on the accelerator, my heart rate up, I think of that visual and sensory image. In my head I croon the word *cooool* over and over and remember the cooling air in my face and the way I felt when I first had this sensation. My foot backs off the accelerator, my heart rate comes down, and I again feel centered rather than the victim of outside forces.

So now I have two powerful images I can summon up to short-circuit stress. One is the visual image of my wife's photo; the other is the physical sensation of coolness on a hot day.

This technique is effective in reducing stress. I strongly recommend it.

CHAPTER 20

Medication

There is a real sense of denial in having this disease. Even after having a heart attack, I still had trouble believing that I needed to take extraordinary measures to control my lipid levels. I resisted taking medications, thinking that exercise and a low-fat diet would turn the tide in my bloodstream. It took several months of near starvation and ever-increasing exercise to understand that all of my efforts were having almost no effect on my blood levels. I still had high cholesterol. I still had low HDL, high LDL, and rising triglycerides.

I had never been one to use medications. I rarely took aspirin, even when experiencing pain. Somewhere deep inside me has always been a fear of putting man-made substances into my body, for fear of side effects yet undiscovered. Now, after a heart attack, I was a walking chemistry set, taking over a half dozen medications every day to regulate my heartbeat, my blood pressure, the clotting ability of my blood, even my stomach acid.

Though I'm not a pharmacist, I've had to become learned about drugs. I am like a constantly shifting science experiment, where my cardiologist and I negotiate each new course of treatment as we monitor my body. I realize there are no absolutes. My condition is not standard, having only recently been identified. My doctor is at the cutting edge of developing treatments for genetically caused heart disease.

I learned early on that this was not like having a broken limb or an ulcer. In those situations, the doctor prescribes specific treatment and the patient follows it. There have been millions of broken limbs and dyspeptic executives, and the medical community, through research over decades, knows exactly how to treat them.

Not so with gene-induced hypercholesteremia and small-particle LDL syndrome. The traditional treatments can be counterproductive. Each patient has to find a comfort level with how aggressive he wants to be in curtailing the disease. Most doctors don't know enough about it to be able to prescribe treatment with the assured outcome as they would with a broken limb or the ulcer.

I surely don't know the entire gamut of treatment options, but I have been at the center of a shifting situation that I hope can shed some light on your own situation.

NIACIN (NICOTINIC ACID)

Reluctantly, I started on drug therapy to control my blood lipids. Adding daily megadoses of niacin was just a small increase in my chemical cocktail. I experienced side effects: flushing, tingling skin, some itching. It took months to go from a very small dose of 100mg/day to a moderately high dose of 3,000 mg/day. Each day, I kept asking myself why I was doing this. Was it really helping?

Niacin works on the liver to increase HDL production. *Never take niacin without a doctor's supervision.* Your liver function must be checked every few months because niacin can cause liver enzyme imbalances and possibly damage. However, if your body can handle it, niacin is an effective way to reverse one of the biggest components of the HeartStopper's game plan: low HDL.

For all the discussions with my cardiologist, for all my reading about what had happened to me, I remained skeptical about the effects of drug therapy until I saw my blood results two months after starting on niacin. My lipid panel showed a dramatic increase in HDL, from 32 to 43. Within six months, my HDL would top out at 52, well above our target of 45. This one therapy lowered my cholesterol/HDL ratio from over 8:1 down to 4.7:1, almost normal. This was convincing evidence that I could counter the effects of the killer gene and possibly avoid another heart attack.

Niacin is a simple, low-priced way to increase HDL and lower triglycerides. The normal recommended daily allowance (RDA) for niacin is 20 mg/day. To affect HDL, one has to ingest about 1,000 mg/day. Normally, this dosage will increase HDL by about 10 to 15 percent. It's possible to take as much as 6,000 mg/day. I went up to 3,000 mg/day and was fortunate to have my HDL go from 32 to 55, a 72 percent increase. I suspect that I got such dramatic results because I started at such a low HDL level.

The single biggest complaint of niacin users is flushing and itchy skin. This occurs when a patient takes too much niacin too fast. One must work up from a minimal dose in slow increments to avoid the side effect of flushing.

The best way to start taking niacin is with 50 mg tablets. Take one at each meal for a total daily dose of 150 mg. Stay on this dose for at least three days. If flushing is minimal, add a 50 mg tablet to each meal for the next plateau of 300 mg/day. Stay on this dosage for at least three days, longer if the flushing persists. If the side effects are too intense, back off the dosage for a few days to maybe 200 mg or 250 mg.

Increasing dosages is more art than science. Anytime the flushing becomes uncomfortable, back off your next dose. The secret is to increase the dosage slowly. This is not a race. If it takes a few months to get to your target dose, so be it. It took me several months to reach 3,000 mg/day.

Once you've reached your target dose, your system will stabilize and you should not experience further flushing, unless you take the niacin on an empty stomach or with coffee or tea. It should always be taken with food.

Another consideration is the brand of niacin you use. Though manufacturers will argue this, there is a difference in brands. My cardiologist cites chapter and verse on the benefits of using what he and his staff feel is the most effective brand: Squibb. Cheaper brands seem less effective and, according to my cardiologist, may be more likely to cause liver damage. The older brands of sustained-release niacin seem most likely to cause liver damage. It pays to spend a little more on Squibb. (I'm not being paid to say this.) My cardiologist recounted numerous cases where patients saw decreases in their HDL levels when they changed brands away from Squibb. When those same patients went back to using Squibb at the same dosages, their HDL values increased.

A long-term niacin side effect I experienced was discoloration of the skin under my arms and in my groin, a condition known as *acanthosis nigricans.* There was no discomfort, but the skin became dark brown and thickened. This is a rare symptom.

As if my emotional roller coaster needed further shocks, my internist freaked when he saw the skin discoloration. It is also the symptom of a rare form of intestinal cancer. I really needed to hear this. Not only was I cursed with a damaged heart, but now I could worry about having cancer, too?

My internist conferred with my cardiologist and we stopped my niacin therapy. Within a month, the discolored skin flaked off. I was gratified to find I did not have a rare cancer, just rare side effects from niacin.

We decided to change my therapy again. I started on a cholesterol-reducing drug with a much smaller dose of niacin (1,000 mg/day). While off niacin, my HDL dropped from 52 to 32. When I resumed niacin at the lower dose along with a cholesterol-reducing drug (known as a statin), my HDL rose to 49, a good number. But even more favorable, the two drugs in combination brought my total cholesterol down to 181, my LDL to 114, and my triglycerides to 113. These were the kinds of levels I had been struggling and experimenting to reach for more than a year. This was a dramatic difference from earlier levels and shows the benefit of experimentation. Not only was my liver less likely to be stressed with the much lower niacin dose, but I didn't reexperience skin discoloration. There are obviously synergies involved with some drugs in combination.

Notably, when I used only niacin, my heart risk ratio was 4.7:1. Taking a cholesterol-reducing drug and niacin together, on the same diet and same exercise regimen, my ratio dropped to 3.8, a much more favorable number. At this point, my cardiologist didn't think I needed to do anything else. After more than a year of trial and error, I was now on a stable drug therapy that had my blood levels in the ideal target range my cardiologist had set for me at the beginning of my therapy.

COUMADIN

Coumadin is a blood thinner. It prevents clotting. It was prescribed to me because of the damaged mitral valve that was causing blood regurgitation within my heart. That extra swirling inside my heart could allow microscopic blood clots to form. Coumadin is effective at preventing these clots inside the heart. Aspirin is not as effective in this application.

My cardiologist pointed out that by taking both aspirin and Coumadin, I was blocking two out of the three chemical ways the body has to create blood clots. This caused my cardiologist some concern. If I was in a severe accident, I could bleed to death before getting to a hospital.

Now, when you are worried about throwing a clot versus having another heart attack, the vague prospect of an accident is not alarming. With my blood levels still in a dangerous range, Coumadin seemed like a small risk to take for a large gain.

Most patients are not on Coumadin more than six months. Because of the bleeding risk, doctors like to get patients off Coumadin once their conditions have stabilized. When that day came for me, I balked. My reasoning was that most post-heart-attack patients did not have mitral valve regurgitation. Though they might take aspirin to prevent clotting in their arteries, aspirin was not the best choice to prevent clotting inside the heart.

At the time, my blood levels had not moved into the range of normal risk. Since I could still be forming cholesterol plaque and since it could tear and cause a clot to form, I was not eager to discontinue Coumadin. My cardiologist tried to persuade me, but I could see no rationale for his advice other than the long-term bleeding risk. Coumadin plus aspirin felt like a force field around me, protecting me from harm.

"I'm not comfortable going off Coumadin yet," I told Dr. Carrea.

"I could just not renew your prescription." It was a hollow threat. He didn't say it with a lot of conviction.

With a grin I said, "Doc, you wouldn't do that."

Pulling his pad in front of him, he drew a quick graph. He was always drawing me pictures of my heart, my arteries, writing down terms. "Okay, your risk on Coumadin is about three percent a year. Project this out for ten years and you have a thirty percent risk of having a bad bleeding incident. If you form a stomach ulcer, you have problems." He drew another set of figures. "On the other hand, your risk of throwing a clot and having a stroke is about one to one and a half percent a year, just a little above normal." He projected these numbers out over ten years. "See the big difference in risk over time? You shouldn't stay on Coumadin for too long."

"I see that. I'll tell you what . . ." This was my prelude for a deal. He settled into his chair. He was used to my horse-trading. There seemed to be no end of things to negotiate. "My cholesterol and LDLs and triglycerides are still too high. When we get those down to normal risk levels, I'll go off Coumadin. That way I'm not likely to throw a clot. This would make me a lot more comfortable. But now while I'm still in danger, I want to stay on it."

"You're not really at that much risk."

"Well, I feel like I am. I don't want to walk around scared. Coumadin is a security blanket for me right now."

"I can buy that. Okay."

It would be six more months before I would feel comfortable going off Coumadin. My blood levels were all in the target range. I was in good health and felt that I was in control of my treatment. I had survived the first year, the year that I had thought of as holding a 5 to 15 percent chance of death. I was now forty-six. How far could I go?

ASPIRIN THERAPY

I take an aspirin every morning. Not for a headache, but to protect my heart. If you think about the big danger of the Heart-Stopper Effect—a sudden, massive blood clot that brings on a heart attack—you can see that there are two components to neutralizing the effect. First, you have to make it difficult for a clot to form. Daily aspirin does this by making blood platelets, the components that form clots, more slippery so that they are less likely to clump together. Second, you have to take away the reason for a blood clot to form. You must cause unstable plaque to convert to stable plaque by starving it of the building blocks of small-particle LDL and triglycerides. This is accomplished through diet, exercise, and niacin therapy.

Aspirin is an important preventive. Studies have shown that for people who have already had one heart attack, aspirin cuts the incidence of a second heart attack by half. If you have heart disease but have not yet had a heart attack, aspirin can increase your chances of not having one. Some doctors have recommended that all men over forty take a daily aspirin whether they have heart disease symptoms or not. Considering that 45 percent of men have no heart disease symptoms before having a heart attack, I am inclined to agree with this advice.

Because aspirin will irritate your stomach and with long-term use can cause stomach ulcers, it's important to use a coated aspirin called *enteric* aspirin. The coating does not dissolve until the aspirin has passed through your stomach and is in your small intestine, where it does no harm. Recognize that because of the coating, enteric aspirin does not go into your bloodstream as quickly as regular uncoated aspirin. Enteric aspirin is not a good choice for quick pain relief.

If you are on aspirin therapy, you should not take more aspirin for pain because more aspirin makes clotting even more difficult. If you are cut or injured, you could hemorrhage. Use acetaminophen for pain or swelling.

In addition to coated enteric aspirin, you should always have a supply of uncoated, regular aspirin around the house, in your car, and at work. If you begin to experience chest pain, you should take two aspirins immediately. If a clot is forming and blocking a coronary artery, an immediate aspirin dose will slow down its growth. In this case, you can see that you want the aspirin to get into your bloodstream as quickly as possible; you don't want coated aspirin for this.

Medication

BLOOD PRESSURE DRUGS

Drugs to lower blood pressure have been around for years. This is part of the regimen with which doctors are comfortable. It addresses one part of the cardiac problem and they know the results they can expect.

If you've had heart damage from a heart attack, part of your heart has "died." Doctors use this term, but in reality, the tissue is not dead. It just doesn't perform as muscle tissue anymore. It has become scar tissue.

If you examine your knees, you will probably find the remnants of childhood skinnings, now faint. These old scars are spread over more area than originally. They are not quite the same tissue as the surrounding skin.

A similar thing happens with heart tissue. Under far more stress than skin tissue, heart tissue also stretches after scarring from an MI. This stretching is dangerous. The larger the heart becomes, the less efficiently it pumps. At some point, it becomes unable to perform sufficiently to keep the body's fluids moving, and congestive heart failure occurs.

When this happens, the lungs and other tissues fill with fluid. Eventually, the heart cannot keep up and the patient has only three options: heart transplant, experimental surgery to reduce the heart's size, or death. None of these options is pleasant to consider.

For this reason, the best course of prevention is to keep the patient's blood pressure as low as possible consistent with daily functioning. By reducing pressures within the heart, stretching of the heart's scar tissues is minimized. The longer that stretching can be forestalled, the longer the patient can enjoy a normal or near-normal existence.

Now the trade-offs. Since the alternative is too grim to argue, patients accept the blood-pressure-lowering treatment. What about the side effects?

First, if you've normally had a blood pressure around 130/80 and it is now brought down to 90/60 (my experience), you will almost surely experience two effects: more fatigue, particularly in the middle of the day, and occasional dizziness when standing up quickly. Also, a hot bath or shower, which normally lowers blood pressure because blood vessels expand when one is hot, may cause dizziness.

Considering the alternatives, these side effects are manageable. Now to the tough stuff. Sex.

Most men experience occasional to frequent impotence under these medications. Here the variables are enormous. How much plaque has built up in the patient's blood vessels? How old is the patient? How much heart damage?

Let's examine a few of these factors. First, most men don't realize that the same cholesterol-rich diet that gave them blockage in their coronary arteries also deposits plaque in other parts of the body. The male penis has less than 1 percent of the blood flow when flaccid than when erect. And, for most of us, that's 99 percent of the time. This means that the blood flow in the penis is small during most of our lives. It is the perfect place for plaque buildup. So, the same forces that give us a heart attack can cause impotence. If the blood vessels can't supply the engorgement necessary for erection, impotence results.

I personally believe that it is not always the blood pressure drugs that cause impotence, but may be rather the cumulative effect of plaque buildup over years made worse by the drugs. I'm not a medical researcher, of course, so this is my own speculation.

What's important here is that it's imperative to keep blood flowing through the arteries of the penis. The old adage "If you don't use it, you lose it" is true in this case. However, many heart patients are fearful of sex, thinking it can bring on a heart attack.

I mentioned earlier the research findings that suggested that the likelihood of a heart attack victim dying from making love was less than one chance in 2 million. The myth is out there, but it's simply not true.

A regular, fulfilling love life is probably one of the best therapies for a heart attack victim. It's good exercise, and the emotional fulfillment does more for the body and mind than a hundred prescriptions.

Not all the blood pressure medications have exactly the same effects. It pays to change prescriptions if impotence becomes a problem. Also, look at the time of day you take the medication. If you normally enjoy lovemaking in the evening, take your medication in the morning. Also look at other medications you may be using. My doctor gave me a mild tranquilizer, Lorazepam, for use if I feel anxious during the day. This medication also makes me drowsy. I sometimes take it in the evening if I'm keyed up and have difficulty sleeping. Add the tranquilizer to the blood pressure medication and Don Juan can become El Zero. So, it's important to plan ahead.

BETA-BLOCKERS

Another key treatment medication is the beta-blocker. These drugs slow the heartbeat and make the heart function more efficiently. Under stress or when exercising, the heart normally speeds up. Beta-blockers prevent the heart from racing and getting out of control. Very fast heartbeats are not efficient pumps. As the damaged heart beats faster and becomes less efficient, it speeds up even more to try to make up for the lack of increased blood flow. It's a vicious cycle that the beta-blocker stops. Otherwise, it's possible to accelerate into all sorts of dangerous arrhythmias.

I will be on a beta-blocker for the rest of my life. It has little effect on most functions, but it does lower blood pressure. So, taking a beta-blocker at the same time one takes blood pressure medication produces a double whammy. Solution: I take the blood pressure medication in the morning and the beta-blocker in the evening to space out the effect. Otherwise, I might find myself drowsy all day.

One possible negative to using beta-blockers is that they increase triglycerides when taken alone. This means beta-blockers could trigger small-particle LDL production. In my case, since I am also taking a cholesterol-lowering drug, this counters the triglyceride-raising effect of beta-blockers. My triglyceride levels are usually below the crossover point for small-particle production; I seem to have found the right balance. However, if you need beta-blockers, you should discuss this issue in detail with your doctor and have your LDL subclass checked until you are sure the beta-blocker is not triggering small-particle LDL production.

VITAMINS AND MINERALS

There is growing evidence of the protective effects of certain vitamins for those of us with heart disease or those trying to prevent it. Over the past year, my cardiologist has prescribed larger-than-normal dosages of these heart-protecting vitamins: folic acid, and vitamins C, E, and B-complex.

When my cardiologist first recommended I take folic acid (also known as folate), I was perplexed. From my nutrition work with pregnant women, I knew that folic acid was essential for preventing birth defects. I was surprised to find that folic acid also reduces homocysteine levels in the blood, and homocysteine has been shown to increase heart attack risk.

After the damage of my first heart attack, my heart probably does not have sufficient redundancy to survive another. So, my cardiologist is aggressive about prevention. In my case, though my homocysteine level is not high, my cardiologist wants to keep it as low as possible. I now take 1 mg of folic acid per day, which is about two and a half times the recommended dietary allowance. For patients with high homocysteine levels, doses as high as 5 mg per day are prescribed.

To work effectively in reducing homocysteine production, folic acid requires the presence of other B vitamins, especially vitamins B-6 and B-12. For this reason, I also take a B-complex vitamin daily.

Any good brand of B-complex vitamins, taken at the 100 percent of RDA dosage, is sufficient. B vitamins are water soluble, so unless you are chewing them like candy, there is no real danger of overdose; any unused vitamins are excreted through your kidneys. However, in choosing a brand, look for one that contains only B vitamins. Some B-complex pills also contain trace elements and metals such as chromium, iron, and zinc. If you take more than a normal dose, the B vitamins will be excreted from your system while the metals will not. Iron, for example, though an essential dietary element, is dangerous to your liver if taken in large doses.

Remember also that niacin is a B vitamin and is present in any B-complex supplement. If you are on niacin therapy, add the amount of niacin from your B-complex dosage into your overall niacin dosage.

When LDL particles oxidize, they become more sticky and more likely to form plaque on an artery wall. (Chemically, oxidation means that a molecule picks up another oxygen atom.) Vitamin E is a strong antioxidant and slows down or prevents this disease process. My cardiologist recommends that I take 800 units of vitamin E daily, which is about twenty-six times the recommended dietary allowance.

Vitamin E is fat soluble, meaning that it dissolves in fat and is moved by the fat-management mechanisms of the body. Consequently, one dose per day is sufficient since it stays in the body much longer than water-soluble vitamins.

Vitamin C is also an antioxidant that helps limit plaque production. It also assists vitamin E in its work. Vitamin C helps keep vitamin E from oxidizing and becoming ineffective. The two together are more powerful than one or the other alone.

Vitamin C is water soluble. A dose you take at breakfast has largely been excreted from your system by lunchtime. So, for vitamin C to remain at therapeutic levels throughout the day, it is important to take it several times during the day. I take 500 mg three times a day for a total of 1,500 mg. This is roughly twenty-five times the recommended dietary allowance.

Potassium is a mineral that is very important to heart functioning. It affects the timing and the efficiency of heartbeats. A potassium level that is too high can cause sudden cardiac death. If it is too low, it can cause arrhythmias and PVCs. For some reason, my normal blood potassium level hovers near the lowest limit of normal. In the hospital, right after my heart attack, when I was experiencing the most PVCs, I was put on a potassium supplement. The PVCs didn't go away, but they did diminish. Ever since, I have taken 25 mEq a day

Because vitamin and mineral doses above the recommended dietary allowance are not always safe and can cause side effects, *always* consult your physician before starting vitamin or mineral therapy.

COLESTID

When it comes to side effects, it seems I have had the rarest and worst. My experience with Colestid was no exception.

This product is designed to absorb bile acids in the intestine and force the liver to draw down LDL to make more bile acids. In this way it reduces LDL levels in the blood.

Colestid is a finely ground resin powder. The treatment is purely mechanical; Colestid does not enter the bloodstream. My doctor thought this might be a good approach since at the time I was taking half a dozen other drugs and we didn't want to increase the chance of interactions.

Within a month of taking Colestid, my LDL level dropped nicely. Apart from occasional gastric discomfort, I was tolerating this new treatment well. We were getting the desired results.

However, Colestid has one rare side effect. Because Colestid changes the chemical balances in the liver, it can cause a slight shift in the acidity of the liver bile, which flows into the gallbladder. This slight change in concentration and acidity can cause gallstones. In my case this is exactly what happened, causing a chain of painful and unfortunate incidents.

CHOLESTEROL-LOWERING DRUGS

I take the minimum dosage of a drug in a group called statins. For almost a year I had resisted starting such drugs for fear of additional side effects and because I could not accept that with all I was doing, I still might need another drug. But I did. No amount of exercise and good eating seemed to be enough to counter the effects of the HeartStopper gene.

The results were startling. Niacin had helped improve my ratio of total cholesterol to HDL and had reduced my LDL level, but the statin seemed to work in a synergistic way with niacin to create much better results. Consequently, I reduced my niacin dose from 3,000 mg/day to 1,000 mg/day. My next lipid panel was encouraging. (Recognize that not everyone will have the same results.)

MY BLOOD VALUES WITH 1,000 Mg NIACIN, 20 Mg STATIN (10/16/98)

Total Cholesterol	High Density Lipoproteins (HDL)	Low Density Lipoproteins (LDL)	Triglycerides
164	45	90	144

Cholesterol/HDL ratio =3.6:1 (risky)

This represented a cholesterol/HDL ratio of 3.6:1, exactly in the normal risk range between 3:1 and 4:1 that my cardiologist set as our goal. Remember my cardiologist's other goals for me? Total cholesterol under 200; LDL under 100; triglycerides under 100; HDL above 45? As you can see from the chart, I was close enough to all those targets to think I had just about the right mix of medication, diet, and exercise.

Most significant were the drops in total blood cholesterol and LDL. There was about a hundred-point drop in both from pre-heart-attack levels. It's the difference between being at the mercy of a killer gene and holding it at bay.

Cholesterol-reducing statins may affect liver function. As with niacin, it is important to be under a doctor's care and to have periodic tests of liver function to make sure the statin is not causing damage.

Because statins are a relatively new class of drugs, there are no long-term studies on their side effects. There have been some concerns that statins might increase the risk of cancer. However, recent studies do not appear to confirm this. Since I will be on this drug the rest of my life, I will closely monitor the results of statin studies as they are released.

You may notice that my triglyceride level was 144, just at the threshold of the range that normally triggers small-particle LDL production. I thought this was an aberration caused by my little binge of sweets the week before my blood test. (Yes, I got caught.) My cardiologist did not believe this short-term rise in triglycerides was causing a small-particle LDL increase because of the dramatic drop in total cholesterol and because my LDL level was relatively low. The building blocks didn't seem to be there. However, we planned to repeat the LDL subclass test in the near future to determine more closely the killer gene's effects at my improved lipid levels. It had been two years since my first small-particle test; using that as baseline data, we thought it would be informative to see what the HeartStopper gene was doing at the molecular level and whether my current regimen had stopped it in its tracks or whether we had to increase my niacin dose.

Because the October 16, 1998, lipid panel looked so good, we discounted the triglyceride of 144. I was so easy to attribute this borderline value to my diet of the previous week.

We were so confident.

Dr. Carrea and I would not learn until three months later that we had made a serious mistake.

CHAPTER 21

Medical Myopia

We spend half our waking hours at work. For many, work is one of the most demanding parts of existence. A heart attack brings one's professional life to a screeching halt.

Following a heart attack, unless one is completely debilitated, one must face the prospect of returning to work, perhaps eagerly, perhaps with trepidation.

It was the last thing I thought about, but the workplace was to confront me with a series of challenges and surprises.

At the time of the heart attack, I was living in Des Moines, Iowa. I worked as a bureau chief in the state health department. I had already given notice to take a job in Nevada and was selling my house and making moving arrangements. My near-fatal heart attack occurred only a few weeks before I was to move.

Once I had the heart attack, my move was put on hold indefinitely until I could undergo rehabilitation and assess what condition I would be in. I was a man in the middle. In those first weeks after the attack, I had no idea if I could regain sufficient strength and ability to return to work. This was a terrifying thought to someone who had worked his way through college, had seldom been unemployed, and who had always been self-sufficient. I had never considered what it might be like to have no income and to become dependent on relatives. It was almost as scary as death.

Some of my coworkers suggested I stay in Iowa. They were supportive. I was amazed at how they rallied around me. For example, my boss, Mary Weaver, a division director, personally chauffeured my out-of-town family around Des Moines until they could pick up my car and settle into my house. Coworkers prepared food and brought it to my house so that my family wouldn't have to worry about cooking, considering the long hours they were spending at the hospital. I was inundated with cards, flowers, gifts, and telephone calls.

Most remarkably, people throughout the health department anonymously donated their annual leave to me so that I would not miss a paycheck after I had used all my own leave. This amounted to many thousands of dollars over the time I was out of work. Their contributions lifted a huge burden from my shoulders. I am forever in their debt.

There was never a question that my employers valued my work and would make whatever accommodations were necessary if I chose to stay in Iowa. I thought this was the norm. I had no idea.

Over the next two months, I regained strength and felt I could go back to work. I rescheduled the movers and signed the final papers on my house sale. My new employers in Carson City, Nevada, had held the job open for me. I couldn't turn back.

When moving day arrived, the movers loaded their truck and departed. My brother, Greg, and my soon-to-be-stepson, Sam, hopped into my car for the 1,600-mile cross-country drive to Reno, Nevada, my new home. Beverly and I then headed for the airport.

During the flight to Dallas I became dizzy due to the reduced cabin pressure and I required on-board oxygen. I learned that airlines pressurize airplane cabins to simulate altitudes of between seven thousand and ten thousand feet. Anyone who's traveled from sea level to a place like Denver knows that the high altitude can have a profound effect on physical activity. Here I was traveling in an airplane that was pressurized to simulate an altitude higher than Denver's. I had not yet achieved sufficient strength to handle this. The American Airlines flight crew requested an emergency landing at Dallas. Soon, we were on the ground and at the center of a small storm of emergency medical technicians and airline staff. American wisely wanted me checked out at a nearby hospital before continuing my trip. I was glad to oblige.

After almost a full day of testing and evaluation, the ER staff declared me okay to continue. Beverly and I returned to the airport, where American graciously put us in first class for the flight to Reno. The competent, professional response by American Airlines and the Dallas airport staff was very reassuring and made me realize that airlines have a lot more behind-the-scenes emergency training than we normally assume. Within a week, I started my new job.

The workplace offers special challenges. How much do you want coworkers to know about your condition? On one hand, do you want strangers to be privy to personal information about your medical condition? On the other hand, it's important for them to know that if you pass out or fall down, it's not low blood sugar; they need to call 911 immediately. For one's own safety, it makes sense to clue in other employees.

Even though I looked fine, was alert, and was capable of doing my job, I didn't realize I was pushing up against the edge of "disability." Technically, under the Americans with Disabilities Act (ADA), I had a disability. Also, having had a heart attack, I had a preexisting condition and could not immediately be covered under my new employer's health plan. I wound up having to buy COBRA coverage from my previous job to tide me over until I was eligible for insurance in Nevada. That was the least of my worries.

Nobody was threatening my job, so I was not being confronted with ADA issues. But I didn't realize that the perception of my health was an issue for my employers.

This may seem far afield, but bear with me. There are two kinds of patients: compliant and noncompliant. Noncompliant patients ignore physical problems and tough it out. For a cardiac patient, this can be fatal. The morgues are full of men who were too proud to admit they were having chest pain and who didn't want to seem like sissies by running to the hospital.

I am a very compliant cardiac patient. My doctors frequently told me that if I experienced anything like the pain I had had during the heart attack, I was to get to a hospital. They advised that if I had any unusual symptoms, I shouldn't take chances. Their message was clear: I should err on the cautious side; that's what emergency rooms are for.

So, ten months into my new job, I felt dizzy one afternoon. I called my wife to tell her what I was experiencing, we conferred, and she called an ambulance. Within minutes, I was on the way to the hospital, my coworkers left behind with stunned looks on their faces.

I was being cautious. I was following my cardiologist's advice. I had no idea how my ambulance ride was being perceived.

A week later, and almost exactly a year after my heart attack, I felt a hot pressure in my chest. It slowly grew until I was on all fours to relieve the gnawing pain. It was familiar, yet not the same as the heart attack pain. With my wife giving me moral support, I endured it for a few minutes and then took a nitroglycerin pill. Within minutes, the pain disappeared and did not return. The next day I called my cardiologist and told him what had happened. Hovering near the anniversary of my heart attack, this episode was chilling to me.

Though I carried nitroglycerin with me at all times, I seldom used it. So, I was terrified that suddenly I needed what I thought of as my "last resort" medicine. However, I learned that my cardiologist expected patients to have occasional pain. That it was relieved by the nitro was what he expected. He was not alarmed and told me not to be.

A week later, the same pain hit me again. I had just come home from work and I was alone. The echoes of that horrid night alone with my heart attack gripped me. I took a nitro pill earlier this time, but to no avail. I took another, and still the pain was growing. In a panic, I dialed 911. Eight minutes later, the ambulance arrived and I was whisked to Washoe Medical Center. En route, they gave me morphine. The pain subsided in a minute.

This perplexed the attending physician. A true heart attack is only slightly buffered by morphine. Morphine takes excruciating pain and converts it to horrendous pain, no better. They ran an EKG in the ER, but my heart did not look out of its normal status. To be safe, they admitted me for observation overnight. In the morning, I felt fine. My heart enzymes were normal, meaning I had not had any heart damage. They released me.

A couple weeks later, I visited the ER near my office, suffering from vague pain and dizziness. What was wrong? It didn't make sense.

Finally, on June 9, 1997, I had such a severe attack of pain at work, I was thrown to the floor. I took four nitros to no effect. I called 911 in a frenzy. The nurses who work in our office checked my vital signs and kept me calm until the ambulance crew whisked me away. I was sure this time I was doomed.

In the ambulance, the EMTs gave me nitro spray under my tongue. Inside two minutes, my pain was gone.

At the ER, they could again find nothing evidently wrong. But to be safe, they decided to transfer me to Washoe Medical Center, which was equipped to perform angioplasty if I needed it. My history was not to be messed with. Angioplasty had saved my life a year earlier.

In the ambulance, as I was being transported from Carson City to Reno, my mind was a maelstrom of concern. Was this the 85 to 95 percent survival odds going against me? Was I dying? Had my heart finally had enough?

This was my fourth trip to the ER. I was admitted to the hospital overnight. They wanted to find out what was causing my recurring problems. One day stretched to two. It took two days in the hospital for the doctors to determine that I had gall stones. The excruciating bouts of pain I had experienced were caused each time I passed a stone.

How could gallstones be mistaken for a heart attack? I recently talked to a woman who'd had her gallbladder removed. She told me that passing a gallstone was more painful than giving birth. I believe her. It's almost more painful than a heart attack.

Two days off had stretched into a week, then two. When I returned home, my wife gave me a letter that she had not wanted to burden me with in the hospital. It was from my boss. It read: *In the past two months you have had several trips to the emergency room. Are you capable of performing the essential functions of your job? Please have your doctor read over your enclosed job description and verify if you can continue working.*

I was suddenly on the razor's edge. My boss was questioning my ability to work. She had written the letter on the same afternoon the ambulance had taken me away from the office. Without yet knowing what my condition was, she had acquiesced to whatever gremlins of doubt had consumed her for the previous few weeks. Without knowing yet that my problem was my gallbladder, she assumed it was heart-related. I was amazed at the lack of compassion she showed by throwing my livelihood into question at a time when I could least deal with it, when such concerns could do the most damage to my frame of mind. Couldn't she have waited a couple days to see what was wrong with me? What a striking contrast this was from the solid, unequivocal support my employers in Iowa had shown me. The letter was shocking.

When I showed the letter to my cardiologist, he was mortified. He apologized for not having picked up on the gallbladder problem earlier, thinking my ailment was cardiac-related. Dr. Carrea immediately saw the connection between his oversight, my ambulance rides, and my employer now asking him if I could continue working. He wrote the required letter, giving all assurances that I was in good health and explaining the gallbladder complication. But nothing could undo the perception that I was physically precarious and possibly not up to working.

This hospital stay required me to use up all of my sick leave and vacation leave. But I had the leave to take. I took no time beyond what I was entitled to. Yet I was now perceived as a walking health risk, one who could unexpectedly miss work, the ultimate sin in the highly regimented organization for which I worked.

I offer this story because it shows the width of the spectrum of response one may encounter. At one end one may find sympathy and support over having a life-threatening disease; the employer is willing to work out whatever is needed to make it possible for an employee to continue. At the other end of the spectrum one may find a more calloused employer who views one as handicapped and possibly incapable of performing one's job properly.

So, how does one handle this? By being compliant with a doctor's recommendations, by being willing to go to the ER when something out of the ordinary happens, it's possible to bring on retribution. Yet if one ignores danger signals or is secretive about a cardiac condition, one threatens one's health.

My advice is to never compromise your health. If you need to go to an emergency room, go. If an employer thinks you are unfit for a job, he or she has to prove that you cannot perform the requirements of the job. Employers are required by the ADA to make reasonable accommodations that would allow you to continue.

So maybe you get a little aggravation from an unsympathetic employer once in a while. Big deal. It's not worth trying to hide your condition. Imagine if nobody in your workplace knew you had a heart condition and you collapsed at your desk one afternoon and everyone who walked by your door thought you were napping. You might be left until you started to stink up the office.

If you have a physically demanding job and a heart attack renders you unable to do it, you'll probably have to change jobs. Maybe your employer will allow you to take over a less demanding position. The employer is not required to do this, but if you are a valued employee, you may be able to work out a satisfactory solution.

In my case, where my job does not require physical exertion, I am not really at risk. As long as my brain works and I can walk in the door in the morning under my own steam, there isn't much a nervous employer can do other than aggravate me with letters. However, in the case of blue-collar workers, a heart attack can require a radical change in jobs, possibly with a significant cut in pay.

There is no doubt this would cause a major life change. At least there is still a life to change. It's a tough break, but so is death.

My advice is, if your job is threatened, learn your rights. Get to a lawyer. But be prepared to make changes and to reassess your career goals.

CHAPTER 22

The Path Not Taken

I saved this story for last. Actually, it is the first part of my story, but until you understood what the HeartStopper Effect is and how it works, until you saw how elusive killer genes can be, you could not appreciate the supreme irony of this final twist in my story.

This is an example of how things can go wrong, of how even highly trained people can miss the killer genes. The price to me is a damaged heart and a shortened life. I hope you do not pay such a price. Read closely. This story took place five weeks before the heart attack that started this book.

On March 30, 1996, at 10:30 P.M. I felt the weirdest, most frightening feeling in my chest I had ever felt. I called an ambulance, something I had never done before. I was not in great pain, but I was jerking, spasming all through my upper torso as if I were getting electric shocks. It was a terrifying experience.

(No, this is not a repeat of the prologue. It sounds incredibly like the heart attack, but it was only the dress rehearsal. This is a wholly different event.)

I was admitted to Mercy Hospital in Des Moines for observation and spent the rest of the night and most of the next morning waiting for test results. I did not sleep.

My thoughts went back, twenty-six years earlier, to when I had held my father and, along with my girlfriend, who was a registered nurse, administered CPR after he collapsed on our kitchen floor. When the ambulance arrived, we refused to give over the CPR to the medics, so they moved my father into the ambulance with my girlfriend and me keeping up our rhythm, she doing compressions on his chest while I did the breathing.

I will never forget the ambulance ride in which my world focused down to my next breath as I forced it through my father's mouth and into his lungs. I will never forget the taste of applejack that was in his mouth. He had come home from work exhausted and had poured himself a small glass of brandy to calm his nerves.

All during that ambulance ride we worked. I had no idea that it was a hopeless task, that he was probably dead only moments after hitting the floor. Cause? A massive myocardial infarction. He never knew he was carrying a killer gene. Nobody knew the HeartStopper Effect existed in 1970.

On March 30, 1996, I also did not know I carried this deadly piece of DNA. On March 30, all I could think of was the remembered horror of breathing into a dead man with whom I would never speak again, though at the age of twenty, there seemed so much more I needed to say. That experience was my only brush with heart attack. But it dominated my thoughts all through that long night of March 30 as I waited to hear a verdict on what was happening in my own chest.

A cardiologist had been assigned to me. He was with a prestigious group of cardiologists on staff at Mercy Hospital. In the early afternoon of March 31, 1996, he met with me to go over my test results.

This was my first exposure to cardiac issues. I was completely ignorant. My cardiologist explained to me that when someone has a heart attack, certain enzymes are released into the bloodstream after a few hours. These CPK enzymes are identifiable and measurable. My level of these enzymes was not elevated, meaning I had not had a heart attack the previous night. This was the only thing I heard. *I had not had a heart attack.* I repeated it over and over in my head.

To be safe, he scheduled me for more testing the next day: a cardiac stress test and an echocardiogram. The stress test involved running on a treadmill while hooked up to an electrocardiogram (EKG) to see how my heart functioned. Before and after the test I underwent an echocardiogram. Both tests showed that my heart was functioning normally under stress and at rest. There was no sign of damage.

I did not know then what I know now. My cholesterol was high at 258. My triglycerides were moderately high. My LDL was moderately high and my HDLs were low. My cholesterol/HDL ratio was 5.8:1, a risky number. Looking only at the numbers, it would suggest a patient who needed treatment to lower cholesterol. But because my heart was not believed to be damaged, because I looked trim and physically fit, my cardiologist did not immediately draw the conclusion that might have resulted in treatment. I did not look like an unhealthy person. This was unlucky. Better if I had been overweight. My cardiologist at the time knew nothing of the HeartStopper Effect and did not see the signals my bloodwork was giving.

Only recently, while examining my hospital records from that day, did I notice another diagnostic clue that was unknown at the time. I remember a doctor at Mercy Hospital telling me, "We're looking at a new indicator for heart attack. It's an enzyme called *troponin*. This is all experimental. We think the heart gives off this enzyme when it's damaged. We don't yet know what level of troponin indicates a heart attack, but we think it's some level over three mg/dL."

My blood test showed a troponin level of 1.9. The Mercy doctors did not think this was significant. Recently, when I showed this old lab report to Dr. Carrea, he said, "My God, you had heart damage."

I cannot fault the Mercy doctors. Troponin was an experimental marker at the time. It would be another year before researchers would properly calibrate their troponin results to accurately diagnose heart attack. My level of 1.9 was way over the now recognized limit of .8 as the threshold for heart damage.

Looking back on my March 30, 1996, incident, Dr. Carrea theorized, "You had plaque in your left descending ventricular artery. It must have torn or cracked and you began to form a blood clot. The clot never got large enough to cause a full-scale heart attack. Overnight, it dissolved and you felt normal again. This was your first bout of unstable angina. Left untreated, unstable angina usually results in a heart attack within six weeks."

Five weeks later, the plaque in my left descending ventricular artery would rupture, causing my blood to clot again and to block that same artery. It would starve the front of my heart of oxygen long enough to kill it.

But in early April 1996, because troponin was not yet an accurate indicator of heart damage, because my stress test and echocardiogram looked normal, and because nobody knew to look for HeartStopper genes, I was told that my chest discomfort had been caused by either torn muscles in my chest or stomach acid backing up from my stomach into my lower esophagus. My doctor literally said Mylanta.

For a week, I took a double dose of ibuprofen to eliminate any irritation in my chest muscles. And at the slightest twinge of discomfort anywhere inside my abdomen, I swigged down Mylanta.

There was no follow-up. Supposedly nothing was wrong with me. On May 9, 1996, that assumption would be turned on its head, and only electricity, big jolts of it administered six dozen times, would keep me alive.

The medical model, the thought paradigm upon which doctors function, is based on treating ailments. It is based largely on correcting problems that have already happened. A doctor can treat a broken arm, but he is not well trained to think of ways to prevent arms from being broken. The Mercy Hospital doctors responded to my original distress call to fix damage that might have occurred. They were as relieved as I was that their diagnostics showed that I had not had a heart attack. The normal cardiac-treatment paradigm and the lack of information on the HeartStopper Effect combined to eliminate heart disease as the cause of my chest discomfort.

In several places, I have mentioned how something unconventional was rejected by either doctors or nurses treating me. When I weaned myself off oxygen, for example, nobody had an explanation for why my lungs began clearing of fluids. I tried something different from the normal plan of care and got results that were unexpected. Because my results didn't fit inside the box of conventional wisdom, the results were largely ignored by everyone but me.

The biggest battle faced by carriers of a HeartStopper gene is to change the beliefs of the cardiac nurses and doctors who "know" which treatments work and which ones don't. Because a HeartStopper gene creates such unexpected anomalies in blood chemistry, it is most difficult to get the experts to accept a treatment that is completely counterintuitive and totally different from what they are used to prescribing.

Here are the dangerous existing paradigms contrasted with the new paradigms the HeartStopper Effect forces us to accept:

Old Paradigm	New Paradigm
All heart disease is treated basically the same.	HeartStopper genes require a specialized treatment approach for each patient.
Fat is bad.	Saturated fat is bad. Intake should be cut to near zero; total fat intake should be under 30 percent of calories and should be composed almost entirely of monounsaturated and polyunsaturated fats (good fats).
Total cholesterol under 200 is healthy.	Total cholesterol is meaningless unless one knows the ratio of total cholesterol to HDL, the levels of LDL and triglycerides in the blood, and the amount of small-particle LDL.

For people with a heart-killer gene, it is crucial to always assume we have a problem. Knowing what I do today, seeing poor cholesterol numbers in a fit, healthy-looking patient would be an immediate tip-off to look for the HeartStopper Effect. Someone who looks healthy should not have the cholesterol levels and the cholesterol/HDL ratio I had.

I am unfortunate in that the symptoms of HeartStopper genes were not on the medical radar screen in 1996. Three years later, only a handful of doctors know how to look for the HeartStopper Effect and how to treat it. It will be years before cardiologists and general practitioners change the basis of their diagnoses to include the new, crucial information that is necessary to suspect killer genes. In the meantime, we patients must be alert to their existence.

Outside of the closed labs of universities and the National Institutes of Health, LDL subclass testing for the HeartStopper Effect has not been available to doctors until recently. Labs equipped to measure small-particle LDL are not just scant, they are nonexistent, except for Berkeley HeartLab. Meanwhile, if my doctor's conservative estimate that 10 percent of the population has the HeartStopper Effect is correct, then 150,000 heart attacks a year could be prevented, of which 50,000 would have been fatal.

What does continued ignorance of HeartStopper genes cost us? Look at my own case. The two weeks in the hospital immediately following my heart attack, along with all the procedures, tests, ER care, and follow-up, came to around $60,000. Since May 1996 my medical care has cost close to $100,000.

The HeartStopper Effect can be neutralized for less than $.50 per day in medication, coupled with a healthy diet and exercise.

Let's use some conservative numbers and estimate the total cost of this overlooked disease. Even though there is strong evidence that roughly a third to half of all heart disease is caused by genetics, let's use the small number of 5 percent as our estimate of the number of people who carry a HeartStopper gene. Then of the 1.5 million heart attacks each year, 50,000 people survive a heart attack caused by HeartStoppers. Let's assume their medical bills over the next five years equal mine in only half that time. The medical cost for each batch of victims would be $5 billion in their first five years of survival, or, let's say, a billion dollars per year. And another 50,000 HeartStopper survivors hit the medical system each year. Each batch represents another billion dollars a year.

The American Heart Association estimates that about 17 million Americans are heart attack survivors. Again, estimating that only 5 percent have the HeartStopper Effect, that means about 850,000 HeartStopper survivors still live. Their annual averaged cost of survival is at least $17 billion.

Now throw in lost wages plus the annual economic cost of the

25,000 gene carriers who don't survive their heart attacks. That's at least another $5 billion. So, just using conservative estimates, the HeartStopper Effect costs us $22 billion a year in medical costs and lost productivity.

Thirty years ago, when the nation's annual highway death toll approached 50,000 people, the government began a massive program of improved vehicle safety. The big three automakers squawked at the government's requirement that they put seat belts in cars. But since then, look at the changes in car design, all intended for increased safety: air bags, door reinforcements, roll bars, collapsible steering columns, crush zones, three-point seat belts, antilock brakes. The list is huge. Car manufacturers have spent tens of billions of dollars to research and implement the government's safety agenda. Yet in 1997, 47,000 people died in car crashes.

I wrote this book to get doctors and patients talking about HeartStopper genes. I expect some people in the medical field to argue with me, to challenge me, to call me nuts. That's fine, because the clinical research has been done and the results are no longer subject to opinion. There are subclasses of LDL that are genetically influenced and whose high levels are deadly if left untreated or if treated as straightforward heart disease. This is fact, not opinion.

As early as 1965, research indicated the existence of LDL subclasses. By 1986 this material was appearing in more detail in medical publications. By 1996, dozens of papers in medical journals had not only proved the existence of at least six different genetically caused LDL diseases, but also showed the successful results of treatment. Yet has there been a groundswell to change the standard diagnostics? No. The most aggressive testing is still the blood lipid panel. In a study I mentioned earlier, doctors who actually knew about small-particle LDL syndrome were wrong 21 to 50 percent of the time when they used a lipid panel to try to predict the existence of small-particle LDL syndrome in patients. Obviously, no huge demand from doctors to test for LDL exists or more than just one commercial lab would be offering these tests.

Why is information about the HeartStopper Effect so slow

getting to doctors? It's probably because of the way doctors get most of their new information. We like to believe that doctors are frequently attending medical conferences and reading medical bulletins. Some do, but the majority are just too busy to reach out for information. They wait for information to come to them.

No human being could keep up with all the developments in medicine, so doctors depend on drug companies and medical-equipment manufacturers for most of their new information. This information is product-driven. It is delivered by the drug companies' field sales staff, known as contact sales reps. The sales reps are thick as flies around a doctor's office. They bring free samples, trinkets, and the occasional free tickets to a show or sporting event, all in the hope of getting someone on the doctor's staff to listen to them. Usually they wind up talking to one of the doctor's nurses, but every so often they get face time with the doctor. In the three golden minutes a doctor gives them between patients, they have to make their pitch and catch the doctor's interest. If they succeed, they get to leave behind product samples and some literature that the doctor and his staff will peruse later. In this literature will be copies of studies and research that support the product claims of the manufacturer.

Depending on which sales rep gets to a doctor first, the doctor will get sold on a specific product's benefits and will begin writing prescriptions for that product. Realize that the doctor can write prescriptions for any drug on the market, but he will tend to write prescriptions for products with which he is most familiar. The contact sales rep's job is to make the doctor familiar with his company's products and to keep the doctor happy. Those new Titleist golf balls or matching Cross pen sets keep the sales rep's products on the minds of the doctor and his staff.

Now let's look at the business angle of this environment. For example, the cholesterol-reducing drug I take costs $1.80 per tablet. Niacin costs $.09 per tablet. The most effective way to treat the HeartStopper Effect is with niacin, an over-the-counter drug made by many different companies. How would it be in the sales rep's interest to chat with a doctor about small-particle LDL syndrome and how niacin counteracts it, when the sales rep can't make any money from this conversation? It's in the sales rep's interest to push the cholesterol drug that costs twenty times what niacin costs and which is protected by a patent. His company will make money and the sales rep will get commissions and bonuses.

In this environment, the drug companies have no reason ever to mention to a doctor anything about small-particle LDL syndrome *because they do not sell prescription drugs that can combat it.* The statins they sell to reduce cholesterol have no effect on small-particle LDL.

If doctors are not jumping on the HeartStopper bandwagon, then it's time patients did. Do you think a lipid panel error rate of 21 to 50 percent is acceptable in diagnosing heart disease caused by small-particle LDL syndrome?

The grim fact is that there is not just one kind of heart disease; the standard of practice we have lived with for decades is now obsolete. There are different causes of heart disease, and in about 50 percent of heart patients, these causes are genetic. This requires that doctors tailor a patient's treatment regimen to the specific cause of disease in each patient. LDL Pattern B (what I have) is treated different from homocysteinemia, which is treated different from an abundance of Lp(a), etc.

I would love to see large-scale surveys to determine the percentage of the population who carry HeartStopper genes. I would love to see some major research dollars spent on looking at the physiological mechanisms that trigger the genes' effects. But in the meantime, without knowing all the chemical intricacies involved, we can still treat these genetic diseases and save lives.

What is to be done? For this knowledge to seep through the medical community and to the grassroots level will take years. In the meantime, I have given you some of the warning signals to watch out for. I strongly urge every adult to get a lipid panel blood test and to use the criteria I outline in chapter 6 to identify your potential for having straightforward heart disease or for carrying a HeartStopper gene.

If you have a history of heart attack in your family, especially if the attacks have occurred in your relatives' thirties and forties, you need a thorough cardiac checkup and bloodwork that includes the LDL subclass test. If you have friends or loved ones who are having chest pain, please convince them to get a cardiac workup and at least a blood lipid panel. If you or someone in your family complains of pain in an arm or pressure in the chest or dizziness or shortness of breath, don't wait to see what happens. Don't be embarrassed. Get to an emergency room, call an ambulance. Do something! Ignorance is deadly.

Patients need to make noise about being tested for the metabolic disorders that may be causing their heart disease. If we push enough, then more doctors will get exposed to this information more quickly, and we'll see genetic testing for heart disease become the norm rather than the exotic exception it is now.

I'm optimistic that better and better remedies for this disease will be found. I'm also optimistic that I have found a regimen that works well for me. I'm living proof that the HeartStopper Effect can be successfully treated and its effects reversed. I am fit, I feel good, and I am much more confident about living a couple more decades than I was in the months just after The Night.

If you look at that night from the viewpoint of a statistician, the odds against my survival were staggering. To have come through that nightmare and to be healthy and functional now is truly a miracle. The more I realize the scope of that miracle, the more convinced I am that I survived in part to carry a message to the millions of people who walk around today oblivious to the time bomb ticking away inside their chest. I am determined to show them how to avoid what I went through.

I wish all of you the gift of health, long life, and happiness.

CHAPTER 23

Good News, Bad News

It was just a few weeks before my manuscript was due at my publisher. Wanting to have the most up-to-date information for this book, I had another LDL subclass test done to show where my body was in my fight against the HeartStopper Effect. When I got the phone call from my cardiologist on the results, they were disturbing.

For the past year I have been on a steady diet regimen, have vigorously exercised three or four times a week, and have used a combination of niacin and a statin to control my blood cholesterol. The lipid panel I had done two months ago was good. Total cholesterol, HDL, and LDL were all low. My triglycerides were above the goal of 100, but didn't seem that far out of whack. All in all, I had been feeling that I had the Type B LDL Pattern licked.

Oh, when will I learn that complacency can kill me?

The recent test was a repeat of the test two years ago that identified that I had abundant small LDL particles (Type B). I wanted to confirm at the molecular level what I thought my past several lipid panels were indicating at the overview level.

The LDL subclass test catalogs the various types of LDL by size and distribution. Basically, we are interested in three gross categories of LDL size: small (very dangerous), intermediate (less dangerous), and large (normally dangerous). The amount of small particles should be under 15 percent.

I expected that my blood test, taken in January 1999, would show that I now had mostly large LDL with very little small LDL. I expected that all the work I had put in over the past two years would have resulted in success.

I was wrong.

My percentages of size distribution were: small, 17 percent; intermediate, 32 percent; and large, 20 percent. (Other subfractions bring the total to 100 percent.) My predominant LDL particle size was intermediate, and my small particles were still too abundant. I was still at more risk of another heart attack than a normal person, and far more than I thought I had been.

It's one thing to experiment on laboratory animals to test one's theories of medicine. Make a mistake and you just order more animals and start over. But when the laboratory in which you test your understanding of a disease is your own body, you have little margin for error.

My first reaction on hearing my results was fear. I could feel a clot forming over some unstable plaque, could feel the pressure in my chest as the artery blocked, knew that I had no redundancy left in my heart and that my mistake was fatal. I was sweating as I set down the phone. I fumbled with my nitroglycerin bottle and shoved a pill under my tongue. It was over. I had failed.

Then I got a grip. There was nothing wrong with me. I had just let disappointment overcome me. My heart was fine. So far.

Then I got angry. I had made two basic mistakes. First, I had used the lipid panels as a proxy for what was happening with my LDL composition. I had assumed as I brought down total cholesterol, LDL, and triglycerides that my LDL subclass was shifting from Type B to Type A. Though by definition I was not the dreaded Type B, I was now almost equally Type A and B. I was straddling the transition point between extreme risk and normal risk.

My own research had shown that lipid panels are good for identifying people with gross cholesterol problems, but that for many carriers of the HeartStopper gene, lipid panel results look normal. The error rate in interpreting Type A or B subclasses from lipid panels is between 21 and 50 percent. I knew this, yet I thought the dramatic downward trend of all my bad blood values would mean a correspondingly dramatic improvement for my LDL subclass. There was improvement, but not anything near what I had expected.

Does this mean a lipid panel is worthless? No. It means that a lipid panel is not a good predictor of Type B LDL subclass in some people. But the lipid panel is still valuable in assessing the effects of diet and exercise on overall blood values. Regardless of the existence of a HeartStopper gene, it should still be everyone's goal to reduce blood triglycerides and LDL while increasing HDL. A lipid panel provides the tool to do this inexpensively and often.

My second mistake was believing that the synergistic effect of taking niacin and a cholesterol-reducing drug would allow me to reduce my niacin dose from 3,000 mg/day to 1,000 mg/day. This reduction was desirable because of the minor side effects I experienced from high-dose niacin. But I now know (after talking to a major drug manufacturer) that cholesterol-reducing drugs do not have an effect on LDL small-particle production. I was wrong to assume that the big cholesterol-reducing effect of the two drugs was reflected in a shift away from small-particle-LDL production at the molecular level.

I thought the problem through and discussed it further with my cardiologist. The solution was fairly simple. I needed to increase my niacin dose. And I needed to get control of a creeping sugar habit that was pushing up my triglycerides. After cutting out all pastries and cookies and brownies two years ago, I had found the pathetic substitute of graham crackers. With tea, these pale proxies gave me the feeling of having a cookie. The sugar content of graham crackers is low, but I was eating too many of them, a package every day.

After the smoke cleared and I had assessed the situation calmly, I was somewhat gratified that what had happened confirmed my research on killer genes. I had proven that sugar triggered triglycerides; these changed LDL production and resulted in the creation of more small and intermediate particles. I had seen firsthand how slightly elevated triglycerides, even in the face of low total cholesterol and low LDL, were a powerful food source for the HeartStopper gene at the molecular level. And just as I had warned others, I now saw that the *only* way to know if I was a normal Type A LDL subclass or a dangerous Type B was to have the LDL subclass test. I could no longer trust a lipid panel, except as a gross indicator of whether my niacin dosage was kicking in.

The day after I received the lab results, I increased my niacin dose and cut out the graham crackers. A month later my lipid panel was the best it had ever been.

MY BLOOD VALUES WITH 1,800 Mg NIACIN, 20 Mg STATIN (3/1/99)

Total Cholesterol	High Density Lipoproteins (HDL)	Low Density Lipoproteins (LDL)	Triglycerides
130	48	67	77

Cholesterol/HDL ratio = 2.7:1 (below average risk)

Three months later I had another LDL subclass test done to see the effects. A distinct shift away from small- and intermediate-particle LDL production toward large-particle production had occurred. I am no longer classed as having an Intermediate LDL subclass pattern. I am now truly Type A. The normal type. Just like everybody else for once.

Further good news. After three years of experimenting to find a stable regimen of diet, exercise, and medication, I wanted to know what had happened at the site where cholesterol plaque had ruptured and caused my heart attack. My blood tests were excellent, but I wanted more tangible proof of what was going on inside me. Was there any new coronary blockage? Had the original blockage grown? I had a nagging fear that the LAD might have closed down and that I might need a stent. So, in September 1999, I had my first angiogram performed since my heart attack. To my pleased amazement, all of my coronary arteries were clear! The site of the original LAD blockage was slightly narrowed, but Dr. Carrea explained to me that this was normal scar tissue and would always be there. He and I were jubilant that the LAD had not closed down. Here was visible, physical proof that we had stopped my killer gene in its tracks. (Remember, even though I appear to have found the proper regimen, treatment of this disease requires individual diagnosis by a cardiologist with a care plan developed specifically for each patient.) These results encouraged me in my wish to live out a normal life span.

I need to celebrate. Maybe just one brownie?

Just kidding.

Epilogue

The LED lights dance on the smoked-glass console in front of me as I adjust the program on the treadmill. The whir of the motor increases and the flexible running belt speeds up. The soft thuds of my jogging shoes echo faintly back from the far reaches of the health club, past the potted palm trees and the stainless-steel water fountain and the shiny chromed weight racks and the espresso lounge. It is late on a Saturday night and all the tonier members of the health club are off at parties and restaurants to show off the bodies they have worked all week to buff and sculpt.

I turn my head and see my reflection in the dark floor-to-ceiling windows that face onto the parking lot. I look fit, but I have no concern for body sculpting or washboard abs. I care not for the latest derriere-hugging, torso-flattering Speedo outfits. I see a reflection in black cutoff sweatpants and a blue, oversize T-shirt spattered with house paint. I see a man pushing beyond a fast walk. I see a man running for his life.

This me is so different from the reflection I saw in a mirror three years ago, when my face was purple and blue and my eyes were swollen, red orbs. I think of that weak creature who could barely stumble across his hospital room. I marvel at how far I've come.

What's different? What's made my survival possible? Yes, the exercise and the medications and the diet are important. But the factor that came before those was knowledge. Without knowledge of the HeartStopper Effect, I would have stayed on the standard heart-attack therapy and I might not be here now. I take no credit for how my feet wound up on this path. It was pure chance. I encountered the right doctors at the right times: the first, a persistent ER cardiologist who would not let me die; the second, a cardiologist who possessed the rare knowledge of the HeartStopper Effect and how to treat it.

I think of how I am now passing this knowledge on to others, like a baton in a relay race. It is a race with a finish line that nobody wants to reach, an endless marathon of survival.

I smile and wave at my reflection. The mirror image waves back.

The journey continues.

Resources

HEART ATTACK WARNING SIGNS
- Crushing chest pain in men; milder in women
- Nausea
- Profuse sweating
- Rapid heartbeat
- Shortness of breath
- Dizziness, weakness, fainting
- Pain in arms, neck, back, jaw, teeth
- Tingling in extremities, especially left arm
- Increased blood pressure

In general, women have milder heart attack symptoms than men. This is mainly because women's hearts are smaller. Women do not usually experience the intense crushing pain that men describe. Many women "just feel bad" when they are having a heart attack. They may have no pain in their left arms, no jaw pain, no crushing feeling in the chest. For these reasons, women frequently do not know they are having heart attacks. They don't go to the hospital; they don't get treatment.

WHAT TO DO IF YOU THINK YOU ARE HAVING A HEART ATTACK
1. Call 911. Do not hang up.
2. Chew and swallow two noncoated, regular aspirin.
3. Lie down in whatever position is most comfortable.
4. Try to relax, try to relax, try to relax.
5. If you have a nitroglycerin prescription, take it while waiting for help.
6. Do not try to drive to the hospital.

Men's symptoms are more dramatic and more easily diagnosed. Men have bigger hearts; they have bigger symptoms. Because of this, it is far more likely for a woman to be sent home from the emergency room with a faulty diagnosis than a man. It is tragic that many of these women go home and die or show up in the ER again hours or days later with more severe symptoms. The heart damage they sustain because of faulty diagnosis could be avoided.

Recently, Jackie Lezzano, a friend I've had since childhood, developed congestive heart failure. For several days she complained of feeling weak and having trouble breathing. She actually went to the hospital, but was not admitted. Her doctor thought she had asthma. He gave her a prescription and told her that in three days she would feel "as good as new." In three days she was dead. She'd had a heart attack. While her heart got weaker and her lungs filled with fluid, she was told over and over that she had nothing wrong with her heart, that her breathing problems were caused by asthma.

Women, be more assertive when you think you are having a heart attack. Demand a troponin test before you allow yourself to be discharged from an ER. Troponin is an enzyme that is emitted by the heart when it is damaged. A troponin test is an accurate indicator of whether someone has had a cardiac event. It is more accurate than the traditional CPK enzymes test that is usually done.

Women, if you think something's wrong with your heart, make the medical professionals who are treating you prove there's *nothing* wrong before they send you on your merry way. The worst that can happen is that you have some unnecessary tests. No, on second thought, the worst that can happen is you *don't* have some unnecessary tests.

CARDIOPULMONARY RESUSCITATION (CPR)

If you have a history of chest pain or have had a heart attack, try to get members of your family to take CPR classes. If your heart should arrest, CPR may be the difference between living and dying. On average, it takes eight minutes for an ambulance to respond to an emergency in the very best rated EMS services. In most cities it takes longer. After four to six minutes without oxygen, brain cells start to die. CPR is the difference between death and survival, brain damage and full recovery.

CPR classes are held at hospitals, health clubs, firehouses, police stations, Red Cross facilities, schools, and other places in your community. Call your local chapter of the American Heart Association or Red Cross to find out where classes are being given near you. If you've already received CPR training, renew your training every two years.

AUTOMATED EXTERNAL DEFIBRILLATORS (AEDs)

For those who have severe heart problems such as arrhythmia, it may be worthwhile to look into buying a portable defibrillator to keep at home. If your heart should stop or go into a deadly rhythm, the defibrillator can shock it back into sync. Today's units contain computer chips that analyze your heart's activity and then calculate the best shock to give it. These units require little training for the person administering the shocks; the unit does all the thinking.

Portable defibrillators cost anywhere from $4,000 up to $20,000. You do not need all the bells and whistles—printouts, monitors, etc.—if you decide to go this route; just get the basic unit.

Even though I have an abnormal heartbeat now, my cardiologist has not recommended that I buy a portable defibrillator. It is not something every heart patient needs; only those with high risk of possible arrest.

One of the newest campaigns being pushed by the American Heart Association is called public access defibrillation. It's been shown that early defibrillation saves lives. The problem has always been in getting a trained person with a defibrillator to the heart attack victim in just a few minutes. In most situations, the victims don't have access to defibrillation until they arrive at the hospital.

But because of computer technology, portable defibrillators require little training to operate. All the calculations for deciding when and how much electrical shock to apply are done by the defibrillator. Even a child can operate one of these units.

It's the American Heart Association's goal to have AEDs available in many parts of a community, such as in office buildings, hotels, shopping malls, and other places where large numbers of people gather; or in rural areas where EMS personnel take longer to arrive. Lay rescuers could apply early defibrillation and save thousands of people every year.

In many cities, firefighters and police carry AEDs. Four airlines that service the United States have begun carrying AEDs on commercial flights: Delta, United, Quantas (Australia), and Varig (Brazil). This list will change, so if you plan to travel and you have concerns about this issue, ask airline reservation agents if their airlines carry AEDs.

The American Heart Association is working to get communities to adopt early defibrillation with AEDs as the standard of care across the country, not in just a few communities.

LDL Subclass and Genetic Blood Testing

In various places in this book I have referred to the need for testing to determine the existence of various apolipoproteins as well as small, dense LDL particles, the markers for the HeartStopper Effect. Your doctor may have an affiliation with a nearby university or research hospital that can perform LDL subclass testing. If not, here's the address of the lab that identified me as a carrier of a HeartStopper gene. Though some commercial labs perform ApoB and lp(a) genetic tests, Berkeley is the only commercial lab in the country that performs the LDL subclass tests that determine LDL particle size. It is run by Dr. Robert Superko, who himself has the HeartStopper Effect.

> Berkeley HeartLab, Inc.
> 1311 Harbor Bay Parkway, Suite 1004
> Alameda, CA 94502
> 800-432-7889

Resources

To get your blood tested, have your doctor order the required shipping package and reagents from Berkeley HeartLab and then have a local laboratory (or your doctor) perform the blood draw. Your local lab will then ship your blood sample to Berkeley via overnight courier. You will have your results usually within two weeks.

THE AMERICAN HEART ASSOCIATION

The AHA has an excellent Web site. I have spent hours there doing research. I have sent questions to its staff via E-mail; the people there respond quickly and have attached reports and references to their responses. AHA's Web address is http://www.amhrt.org.

THE NATIONAL HEART, LUNG, AND BLOOD INSTITUTE

The institute is part of the federal government's National Institutes of Health. The institute has an excellent Web site with interactive features. You can perform diet analysis or determine your heart attack risk by walking through its easy-to-use interactive tools. This is a huge site with resources for the casually curious or the professional. NHLBI's address is http://www.nhlbi.nih/nhlbi/nhlbi.html.

THE HEARTSTOPPER SITE

The address for my personal Web site is www.eatfatbehealthy.com. Information in this book is presented there, as well as updates and links regarding tests for the HeartStopper Effect. For the skeptical doctors who will read my book and say, "Yeah, show me," I have included a medical-publication reference section at the end of this book and will include it on my Web site. I welcome your E-mails and will choose representative questions to answer on the Web site. I hope over time to make this Web site a place where readers of *Eat Fat, Be Healthy* can visit to update their knowledge of cardiac killer genes or to make contributions of their own treatment discoveries.

I have set up links to the American Heart Association and the National Heart, Lung, and Blood Institute and will add other resources as I find them.

References

These are the scientific papers I used when researching this book.

Austin, M. A., J. L. Breslow, C. H. Hennekens, et al. "Low density lipoprotein subclass patterns and risk of myocardial infarction," *Journal of the American Medical Association* 260 (1988): 1917–21.

Austin, M. A., L. Mykkanen, J. Kuusisto, et al. "Prospective study of small LDLs as a risk factor for non-insulin dependent diabetes mellitus in elderly men and women," *Circulation* 92 (1995): 1770–78.

Blankenhorn, D. H., S. P. Azen, D. M. Kramsch, et al. "Coronary angiographic changes with lovastatin therapy," *Annals of Internal Medicine* 119 (1993): 969–76.

Colditz, G. A., E. B. Rimm, E. Giovannucci, et al. "A prospective study of parental history of myocardial infarction and coronary artery disease in men," *American Journal of Cardiology* 67 (1991): 933–38.

Dawber, T. R. *The Framingham Study* (Cambridge, Mass.: Harvard University Press, 1980).

Dreon, D. M., H. Fernstrom, B. Miller, et al. "Low density lipoprotein subclass patterns and lipoprotein response to a reduced-fat diet in men," *FASEB J* 8 (1994): 121–26.

Dreon, D. M., H. Fernstrom, P. T. Williams, et al. "LDL subclass patterns and lipoprotein response to a low-fat, high-carbohydrate diet in women," *Arterioscler Thromb Vasc Biol* 17 (1997): 7007–14.

Dreon, D. M., H. A. Fernstrom, P. T. Williams. "A very low fat diet is not associated with improved lipoprotein profiles in men with a predominance of large, low-density lipoproteins," *Am J Clin Nutr* 69 (1999): 411–18.

Dunn, P., R. Meese, H. R. Superko, et al. "Cardiovascular risk reduction is cost effective in the real world," *Circulation* (1997): (abstr) #4000.

Franceschini, G., M. Cassinotti, G. Vecchio, et al. "Pravastatin effectively lowers LDL cholesterol in familial combined hyperlipidemia without changing LDL subclass pattern," *Arterioscler Thromb* 14 (1994): 1569–75.

Frick, M. H., O. Elo, K. Haapa, et al. "Helsinki Heart Study: Primary-prevention

References

trial with gemfibrozil in middle-aged men with dyslipidemia," *New England Journal of Medicine* 317 (1987): 1237–45.

Friedlander, Y., D. Lev-Merom, and J. D. Kark. "Family history as predictor of incidence of acute myocardial infarction: The Jerusalem Lipid Research Clinic" (paper presented at the 2nd International Conference on Preventive Cardiology and the 29th Annual Meeting of the AHA Council on Epidemiology, Washington, D.C., June 18–22, 1989).

Gardner, C. D., S. P. Fortmann, R. M. Krauss, et al. "Small low density lipoprotein particles are associated with the incidence of coronary artery disease in men and women," *Journal of the American Medical Association* 276 (1996): 875–81.

Genest, J. J., S. S. Martin-Munley, J. R. McNamara, et al. "Familial lipoprotein disorders in patients with premature CAD," *Circulation* 85 (1992): 2025–33.

Goldbourt, U., U. de Faire, and K. Berg. *Genetic Factors in Coronary Heart Disease* (Hingham, Mass.: Kluwer Academic Publishers, 1994).

Hamsten, A., and U. de Faire. "Risk factors for coronary artery disease in families of young men with myocardial infarction," *American Jounal of Cardiology* 59 (1987): 14–19.

Hodis, H. N., and W. J. Mack. "Triglyceride-rich lipoproteins and the progression of coronary artery disease," *Current Opinion in Lipidology* 6 (1995): 209–14.

Hodis, H. N., W. J. Mack, S. P. Azen, et al. "Triglyceride-and-cholesterol-rich lipoproteins have a differential effect on mild/moderate and severe lesion progression as assessed by quantitative coronary angiography in a controlled trial of lovastatin," *Circulation* 90 (1994): 42–49.

Krauss, R. M., and P. J. Blanche. "Detection and quantitation of LDL subfractions," *Current Opinion in Lipidology* 3 (1992): 377–83.

Krauss, R. M., F. T. Lindgren, P. T. Williams, et al. "Intermediate-density lipoproteins and progression of coronary artery disease in hypercholesterolaemic men," *Lancet,* July 11, 1987, 62–65.

Lamarche, B., A. Tchernof, S. Moorjani, et al. "Small, dense low-density lipoprotein particles as a predictor of the risk of ischemic heart disease in men. Prospective results from the Quebec Cardiovascular Study," *Circulation* 95 (1997): 69–75.

Manninen, V., L. Tenkanen, P. Koskinen, et al. "Joint effects of serum triglyceride and LDL cholesterol and HDL cholesterol concentrations on coronary heart disease risk in the Helsinki Heart Study," *Circulation* 85 (1992): 37–45.

Marenberg, M. E., N. Risch, L. F. Berkman, et al. "Genetic susceptibility to death from coronary heart disease in a study of twins," *New England Journal of Medicine* 330 (1994): 1041–46.

Miller, B. D., E. L. Alderman, W. L. Haskell, et al. "Predominance of dense low-density lipoprotein particles predicts angiographic benefit of therapy in

References

the Stanford Coronary Risk Intervention Project," *Circulation* 94 (1996): 2146–53.

Miller, B. D., R. M. Krauss, L. Cashin-Hemphill, et al. "Baseline triglyceride levels predict angiographic benefit of colestipol plus niacin therapy in the Cholesterol-Lowering Atherosclerosis Study (CLAS)," *Circulation* 88 (1993): I-363.

Nishina, P. M., J. P. Johnson, J. K. Naggert, et al. "Linkage of atherogenic lipoprotein phenotype to the low-density lipoprotein receptor locus on the short arm of chromosome 19," *Proceedings of the National Academy of Sciences USA* 89 (1992): 708–12.

Rissanen, A. M. "Familial occurrence of coronary heart disease: Effect of age at diagnosis," *American Jounal of Cardiology* 44 (1979): 60–66.

Rotter, J. I., X. Bu, R. Cantor, et al. "Multilocus genetic determination of LDL particle size in coronary artery disease families," *Clin Res* 42 (abstr) (1994): 16A.

Sacks, F. M., M. A. Pfeffer, L. A. Moye, et al. "The effect of pravastatin on coronary events after myocardial infarction in patients with average cholesterol levels," *New England Journal of Medicine* 335 (1996):1001–9.

Schildkraut, J. M., R. H. Myers, L. A. Cupples, et al. "Coronary risk associated with age and sex of parental heart disease in the Framingham Study," *American Journal of Cardiology* 64 (1989): 555–59.

Stampfer, M. J., R. M. Krauss, P. J. Blanche, et al. "A prospective study of triglyceride level, low density lipoprotein particle diameter, and risk of myocardial infarction," *Journal of the American Medical Association* 276 (1996): 882–88.

Superko, H. R. "New aspects of cardiovascular risk factors including small dense LDL, homocysteinemia, and Lp(a)," *Current Opinion of Cardiology* 10 (1995): 347–54.

———. "Beyond LDL-C reduction," *Circulation* 94 (1996): 2351–54.

———. "Lipid disorders contributing to coronary heart disease—an update," *Current Problems in Cardiology* 21 (1996): 733–80.

———. "What can we learn about dense LDL and lipoprotein particles from clinical trials?" *Current Opinion in Lipidology* 7 (1996): 363–68.

———. "The atherogenic lipoprotein profile," *Science and Medicine* 4 (1997): 36–45.

———. "Small dense LDL: The new coronary artery disease risk factor and how it is changing the treatment of CAD," *Preventive Cardiology,* 1998.

Superko, H. R., P. S. Bachorik, and P. D. Wood. "High-density lipoprotein cholesterol measurements," *Journal of the American Medical Association* 256 (1986): 2714–17.

Superko, H. R., and KOS Investigators. "Effects of nicotinic acid on LDL subclass patterns," *Circulation* 90 (1994): I-504.

Superko, H. R., and R. M. Krauss. "Coronary artery disease regression. Convincing evidence for the benefit of aggressive lipoprotein management," *Circulation* 90 (1994): 1056–69.

———. "Reduction of small dense LDL by gemfibrozil in LDL subclass pattern B," *Circulation* 92 (1995): I-250.

Superko, H. R., P. T. Williams, E. L. Alderman for the Stanford Coronary Risk Intervention Project Investigators. "Differential lipoprotein effects of bile acid binding resin in LDL subclass pattern A versus B," *Circulation* 86 (1992): I-144.

Watts, G. F., S. Mandalia, J. N. Brunt, et al. "Independent associations between plasma lipoprotein subfraction levels and the course of coronary artery disease in the St. Thomas Atherosclerosis Regression Study (STARS)," *Metabolism* 42 (1993): 1461–67.